Strategies to Promote Self-Management of Chronic Disease

American Hospital Association

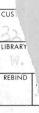

AHA

TM

STRATEGIES TO PROMOTE
SELF-MANAGEMENT OF CHRONIC DISEASE

AHA/CDC Health Education Project*
Center for Health Promotion
American Hospital Association
840 North Lake Shore Drive
Chicago, Illinois 60611

*This project is funded by the U.S. Department of Health and Human Services,
Public Health Service, Centers for Disease Control, Center for Health
Promotion and Education, Community Program Development Division, Atlanta,
Georgia, under contract number 200-79-0916 with the American Hospital
Association, Chicago, Illinois

Library of Congress Cataloging in Publication Data
Main entry under title:

Strategies to promote self management of chronic disease.

   "AHA/CDC Health Education Project, Center for Health
Promotion, American Hospital Association."
   Bibliography: p.
   1. Patient compliance. 2. Self-care, Health.
I. American Hospital Association. Center for Health
Promotion. [DNLM: 1. Self care. 2. Patient education.
W 85 B485]
R726.5.S78 1982   615.5   82-11533
ISBN 0-87258-380-5

AHA-070150

Copyright 1982 by the
American Hospital Association
840 North Lake Shore Drive
Chicago, Illinois 60611

CONTENTS

In order to provide the reader with a context in which to read and appreciate this document, a brief history of its development follows.

In August 1979, the Center for Health Promotion of the American Hospital Association (AHA) was awarded a contract (no. 200-79-0916) by the Center for Health Promotion and Education, Centers for Disease Control, HHS, to improve ambulatory patient and community health education provided in various health care settings.

During the first year of the project, as part of a subcontract, staff of the University of Wisconsin, Center for Health Sciences, were to determine if previously developed staff manuals for teaching patients[1] would be useful for staff in ambulatory care settings; if yes, what revisions, if any, would be needed; and what additional information would be useful for ambulatory care staff.

A structured interview protocol was used to collect information from nurses, pharmacists, nutritionists, physicians, and occupational therapists in hospital outpatient clinics, freestanding clinics, public health departments, arthritis multipurpose centers, diabetes research and training centers, voluntary agency affiliates, and the Indian Health Service.

Recommendations for additional information included the need for resources relating to adherence strategies and chronic disease. In order to respond to this recommendation the document, Strategies to Promote Self Management of Chronic Disease, was written.

---

[1] The manuals are Implementing Patient Education in the Hospital, Staff Manual for Teaching Patients about Hypertension (also staff manuals for teaching patients about chronic obstructive pulmonary disease, diabetes mellitus, and rheumatoid arthritis), the Media Handbook, and Medication Teaching Manual. These are available for purchase through the American Hospital Association.

ACKNOWLEDGMENTS

This book reflects the insights of several individuals who served informally as a sounding board while the book was conceptualized and written. Their experience with individuals with chronic disease and with strategies described in this book stengthened the book considerably. The support and advice of the following individuals is greatly appreciated: Sue Daggett, MSN, Harvard Community Health Cooperative; Karen Eichelberger, MSN, Monona Grove Clinic, Lecturer Nurse Practice program, University of Wisconsin School of Nursing; Jean Espenshade, MSN, Department of Psychology, University of Wisconsin; Marie Heiss, R.N., MS, Clinical Nurse Specialist Rheumatology, Madison; Patricia Angvik Herje, MSN, Director of Health Education, Jackson Clinic, Madison; Sandra Olin Lewis, BSN, Vermont Lung Association, South Burlington; Kathleen Poi, MSN, Assistant Director, University of Wisconsin Health Services, Assistant Clinical Professor, School of Nursing; Sandy Ward, MSN, Clinical Nurse Specialist, Mendota Mental Health Center, Madison; Jean White, MSN, Clinical Nurse Specialist, Adult Primary Care Clinic, University of Wisconsin Hospitals and Clinic. Both Janis Fink, MSN, Washington, D.C. and Roberta Wallace, MA, Associate Director, Area Health Education Center, University of California, Department of Family Medicine, Sacramento, reviewed the entire manuscript and provided extremely helpful suggestions for presenting information in a way that clinicians would find most useful.

I would also like to thank and acknowledge the generosity of Kate Lorig, Ph.D., Stanford University; JoAnn Earp, Ph.D., Univeristy of North Carolina, Chapel Hill; and Susan Steckel, Ph.D., University of Michigan for sharing their prepublication data.

Equally important were the individuals with chronic disease and their families who shared their perspectives of what it is like to live with a chronic condition. Their openness and wisdom is deeply appreciated.

Every book has its unsung heroines and this book has many. Theresa Wadden, MS, did voluminous library research on adherence and self-management literature. A. Frances Lindner, MA, interviewed individuals with chronic disease and provided numerous insights into the realities of having a chronic condition. Without her constant support and organizational skills this book would never have been completed. Gundega Korsts, MA, edited the book. Bonnie Hayward and Mary Weber assisted in typing the manuscript.

Elizabeth Lee, MSN, Center for Health Promotion, American Hospital Association, provided direction and critical feedback throughout this effort. Her commitment to helping clinicians and clients alike made this endeavor possible in the first place.

Lastly, thank you, to Larry and Frances for their patience, support and resourcefulness. No family could have been more understanding or helpful.

Betty Chewning, Ph.D.
Assistant Clinical Professor,
University of Wisconsin,
Center for Health Sciences,
Madison, Wisconsin,
March, 1982.

INTRODUCTION

Effective management of a chronic disease depends upon individuals actively regulating their condition to retard or prevent its deterioration. The question facing a health care professional is how to support and encourage the management of the condition in such a way that the individual feels comfortable enough to return for consultation as management problems arise or as new priorities emerge. More than with an acute condition, management of a chronic condition requires an ongoing working relationship between client, or patient, and provider so that the care plan can be adjusted in response to the client's changing self-awareness, circumstances, and condition.

Unfortunately providers and clients often report more frustration than openness or trust in their working relationship. From the provider's perspective, some clients show little interest in managing their own condition. At times clients seem to resist all efforts by providers to promote management of the chronic condition.

From the client's perspective, working toward self-management can be equally uncomfortable. As one client with chronic obstructive pulmonary disease (COPD) stated:

> "I believe that the nurse and doctor are trying to help when they tell me to do these things, but some of it I just can't do. I just don't think they know what it's like to do these things when you can't breathe."

Or as another client, a young woman with diabetes, said:

> "Each time I saw someone [staff] new, I dreaded it. I thought they'll tell me everything I should be doing and lecture me about anything I'm not doing, like asking me, 'Well, why aren't you doing your urine testing?' So I just started lying. I didn't feel like I could be straight and really get some help."

Clearly something is wrong with efforts to help clients help themselves when providers find the process frustrating and clients fear being honest with providers. The goal of this document is to help providers involve clients successfully in managing their conditions through the selective use of problem solving and adherence strategies. It is hoped that these strategies can make working together a more rewarding process for provider and client alike.

The terms client, adherence, and self-management will be used throughout the book. As Szass and Hollander (1956) point out, the traditional patient role connotes a passive, dependent set of behaviors. Since this document focuses on the potential for increasing the active responsibility of individuals using health care services, the word "client" rather than "patient" will be used. A similar concern led to the decision to use the term "adherence" rather than "compliance." More than compliance, adherence connotes an active partnership between provider and client, a partnership in which both provider and client strive to ensure that the client will become as self sufficient as possible in managing his or her condition. In this context, the client who is adherent is, by a voluntary and active decision, following a regimen that he or she feels is sensible and contributes to management of the condition. The term self-management will be used to emphasize the individual as a decision-maker, one who uses problem-solving skills to deal with issues arising from the regimen and the condition itself. As manager, the client uses knowledge and experience to increase his or her flexibility in applying the principles underlying the medical regimen, rather than only following the specifics of the regimen.

This book draws upon three resources to reach its goal of encouraging active self-management--the insights of clients themselves, research literature on adherence, and the experience and suggestions of providers. The first chapter provides an overview of the self-management strategies discussed in this book and offers a process for using these strategies selectively, given the provider's resources and characteristics of the client population. The second chapter presents the client's perspective of what it is to have and manage a chronic condition. Interviews with 25 clients provide the basis for this chapter. Building on this perspective, the third chapter discusses a joint client and provider process for devising and revising regimens. Because there is growing evidence that more than one type of intervention is necessary to promote self-management, at least for clients with a history of nonadherence, subsequent chapters then discuss specific strategies that can be used to augment the basic one to one process discussed in chapter three.

Strategies discussed in subsequent chapters include contracting, medical record co-authoring, self-monitoring, educational support groups, family involvement, and telephone or postcard contact with clients. While some of these strategies, such as postcard contact, are relatively inexpensive and applicable to a broad range of clients, other strategies (e.g., self-monitoring) are not. Although it is helpful to read the first three foundation chapters first, subsequent chapters on individual strategies can be read in any order. These chapters have been written to stand independently.

To help readers evaluate and use the strategies in chapters 4 through 8, each is discussed in terms of: 1) critical components which influence the strategy's effectiveness; 2) situations and clients for whom the strategy has been shown to have the strongest impact; 3) common client and provider reactions to the strategy; and 4) systems issues, such as resources required to use the strategies effectively. Because literature on some of these topics is scant, provider experience has been an additional source of information. It is hoped this information will help readers apply these strategies selectively and effectively.

Although there is a voluminous literature on adherence, the quality varies widely; therefore, only a few studies are reviewed within the text of each chapter. Studies were selected which:

1) focus on individuals being treated on an outpatient basis for arthritis, COPD, diabetes, or hypertension;

2) examine a strategy to promote self-management;

3) use an outcome measure relevant for adherence; and

4) either meet accepted research standards (control groups, client sample size, reliable outcome measures) or provide particularly interesting qualitative information about the client-provider experience.

To help readers who wish to use a particular strategy, information about how it was used in different studies is available in the annotated bibliography that appears at the end of the book. The annotations include information on the client population studied, the purpose of the study, the study's research design, how the intervention (e.g., contracting) was done, measures used to evaluate the impact of the intervention on adherence (e.g., blood pressure, appointment-keeping rates, self-reported medication adherence), results of the study that have implications for provider practice, and limitations of inference (any aspects of the study that suggest one should be careful about drawing conclusions or generalizing from the study's results). Technical terms used in the annotated bibliography are defined in a glossary that precedes the bibliography.

REFERENCE

1. Szass, T. S., and Hollander, M. V. H. A contribution to the philosophy of medicine. Arch. Intern. Med. 97:585-592, 1956.

CHAPTER 1
A STEP APPROACH TO SELF-MANAGEMENT

Clients with a chronic condition strive to maintain the quality of their lives. For the most part, clients want to be well, to maintain their usual activities and their ability to function normally (Cluff, 1981). It is especially important for health care providers to work with clients and families to establish treatment plans that optimize the client's quality of life and ability to function normally. One of the primary challenges to health providers is finding ways to promote self-management that are sensitive to the individual client's needs and are realistic given the provider's resources. This chapter suggests a process that providers can use to selectively apply strategies discussed in this book so that limited resources are used where they are most needed and can be most effective.

Several assumptions underlie the process to be discussed. First, clients vary in how much help and attention they want and need to manage their conditions effectively. Some clients seem to incorporate self-management into their lives fairly quickly, while others need significantly more support to begin and continue the process. A second assumption is that for the latter group it will be particularly important to consider using a combination of strategies to promote self-management. While regular clinic visits may be sufficient for one client, another may need to have regular telephone contact or small group involvement as well. A third assumption is that clients will have different goals or standards for self-management, with some clients seeking the best control they can possibly have, while others set their goals somewhat lower. Further, clients will vary in their preferences for how to reach their goals. A fourth assumption is that developing a systematic approach toward promoting self-management will lead to more effective results. Therefore it is useful to develop a protocol for assessing and responding to self-management needs of clients in much the same way that medication and other treatment needs are addressed.

The process being suggested is a step approach, similar to the familiar step approach used in drug therapy. Applying the process to an individual client, the provider introduces a first level strategy and evaluates the client's progress in self-management. If the first level strategy is unsuccessful with a client, a second level strategy is then introduced and evaluated. As the first step of designing such a protocol for a client population, providers need to identify a set of strategies that can be used with all clients initially. Second, providers need to identify a subset of more costly interventions which can be used with clients who have a history of poor adherence, who are having problems managing their condition, or who expect to have problems.

In deciding how to structure a step approach for the client population as a whole, begin by assessing client population needs and provider resources. In terms of client needs, ask what is the nature of the client population you see. What are the most common problems in self-management? Are there any problems, such as high missed appointment rates, that are of particular concern? If yes, this information, in addition to population characteristics such as age, types of chronic conditions seen, and literacy level, can help identify level I strategies.

To select strategies which would be realistic given available resources consider the following questions. Is there a team of providers who can work together and if yes, how can their time and skills be used best? Timewise, where does the flexibility lie--are there predictable times during the week when longer visits can be scheduled, either for first-time sessions or for follow-up; are there times during the day or week when telephone contacts can be regularly scheduled; is the client flow such that frequent follow-up visits can be scheduled if necessary? After surveying the available resources, choose a few strategies that seem most feasible. This first level may include combinations of strategies, similar to those discussed in Chapter 3, "Devising and Revising the Regimen" (see Table 1).

TABLE 1. EXAMPLES OF LEVEL I STRATEGIES OFFERED TO ALL CLIENTS

Clinic Visit Schedule	Examples of Strategies
Monthly visits, until condition regulated; bi-monthly visits for monitoring.	-- Identify and use client concerns as source of motivation. -- Tailor regimen to client. -- Educate about condition, seriousness, risks, management, rational for management elements (diet, meds, etc.). -- Monitor quality of life issues and self-management. Listen, problem-solve, elicit feedback. -- Involve family (as client and family desire). -- Consider informal or formal contracts regarding client behaviors.

The selection of Level I strategies will vary with the nature of the client population, the personal preferences of the provider, and the resources of the health care setting. For example, one provider may want to establish an initial teaching visit with all clients, while another provider would do this only rarely. Likewise, some providers may have a client population with high missed-appointment and drop-out rates, and therefore may elect to use postcard appointment reminders as a baseline strategy for all clients.

After determining the baseline strategies to use with all clients, the next step is to identify what indicators the provider will use to assess whether a second level of interventions should be used with a particular client. A variety of studies (Haynes, 1976; Haynes, 1980; Johnson, 1978; Morisky, 1980; Sackett, 1979) suggest that clients need more attention and self-management support who:

-- have a history of nonadherence
-- expect to have trouble remembering their medications
-- have more complex regimens
-- are known to be at risk for complications

Usually client interviews, along with existing medical records and appointment keeping rates, are good sources of this information. Haynes (1980) reports that asking clients directly about their adherence is effective; 75% of the clients in this research were correctly classified as adherent or nonadherent from self-report alone. Thus, an ongoing dialogue between client and provider about adherence progress is useful for evaluating whether a second level of intervention is necessary.

After choosing indicators such as those listed above, the third step in designing a protocol is deciding which interventions can compose Level II, to be introduced after the Level I baseline interventions. Again it will be critical to select strategies that are realistic given the available resources. Chapters 4-8 provide examples of strategies which might be included as options (see Table 2).

TABLE 2. EXAMPLES OF LEVEL II STRATEGIES
OFFERED TO A SUBSET OF CLIENTS

Clinic Visit Schedule	Examples of Strategies	Chapter
Increase frequency of visits to every two weeks.	- Consider simplifying regimen......................3	
	- Assess client priorities, concerns, barriers that may affect self-management.................3	
	- Consider client contracts.........................4	
	- Teach self-monitoring and record keeping skills...5	
	- Consider educational-support groups...............6	
	- Involve family more intensely (if both family and client are willing).........................7	
	- Use reminders (postcards, telephone).............8	

Up to this point Level II strategies have been discussed solely in terms of clients who need additional help to manage their conditions. At times, however, clients who already are managing their conditions effectively will want to take advantage of Level II strategies. For example, if an educational-support group is organized, it is likely that a variety of clients will be interested in joining. The goal in identifying the second level of interventions is to help providers spend their additional resources most appropriately, both on clients who have the greatest need and on those whose motivation is high.

McClellan and Jones (1978) offer a simple example of stepped introduction of strategies. In an outpatient program for clients with hypertension, two-week visits are scheduled for all clients until their blood pressure reaches the goal. During these visits, a nurse clinician reviews the drug program, does patient education, and reinforces the client's self-management efforts. Since this is the basic level of care offered to all clients it can be considered the first level strategy for encouraging self-management. While many clients do fine solely by making the visits every two weeks, a subset of clients do not. For clients who start to miss appointments, a second level of intervention has been devised. If a client misses an appointment, a telephone call or postcard is used to reschedule the appointment and reinforce its importance. Often this is sufficient to keep clients in care. However, a further subset of clients requires a third level of intervention more costly than the preceding pattern of visit and telephone or postcard follow-up. If clients haven't returned for care with these earlier interventions, the provider makes a home visit. In this manner, a series of three-step interventions are made available to clients. Clients' appointment-keeping behavior acts as the primary indicator of whether a more intensive strategy is needed. Sackett an others (1978) propose a similar sequence of strategies for clients with hypertension, with the final step being to teach clients how to measure their blood pressure.

Ultimately, the success of any partnership between client and provider depends upon mutual respect. Thus, the success of using any strategies discussed in this book depends on the quality of client-provider relationship. If trust and openness can be established, both provider and client can help each other toward the common end of better self-management.

To help demonstrate the usefulness of achieving this openness, the following chapter presents the results of interviews with 25 clients. Their perspective, often quite dissimilar from those a provider might have, help to provide a context for the subsequent discussion of individual strategies listed in Tables 1 and 2 above.

REFERENCES

Cluff, L. E. Chronic disease, function and the quality of care. J. of Chronic Dis. 34:299-304, 1981.

Haynes, R. B. A critical review of the "determinants" of patient compliance with therapeutic regimens. In: Sackett, D. L., and Haynes, R. B., editors. Compliance with Therapeutic Regimens. Baltimore: Johns Hopkins Press, 1976, pp. 26-40.

Haynes, R. B., and others. Can simple clinical measurements detect patient non-compliance? Hypertension 2:757-764, Nov. 1980.

Johnson, A. L., and others. Self-recording of blood pressure in the management of hypertension. Can. Med. J. 119:1034-1039, Nov. 1978.

McClellan, W., and others. Prolonged blood pressure control in a rural outpatient hypertension clinic: a description of methodology and results. Presented at National Conference on High Blood Pressure Control, Los Angeles, 1978.

Morisky, D. E., and others. The relative impact of health education for low- and high-risk patients with hypertension. Preventive Med. 9:550-558, 1980.

Sackett, D. L. A compliance practicum for the busy practitioner. In: Haynes, R. B., and others, editors. Compliance in Health Care. Baltimore: Johns Hopkins Press, 1979, pp. 286-294.

Sackett, D.L., and others. Patient compliance with antihyertensive regiments. Patient Counselling and Health Educ. 1:18-21, First Quarter 1978.

CHAPTER 2
THE CLIENT'S PERSPECTIVE

One assumption underlying this book is that a provider who understands a particular client's perspective has a tremendous advantage for helping the client assume a more independent role of self-management. To aid the process of understanding clients, this chapter presents excerpts from 25 client interviews conducted specifically for this book. The interviews were designed to help illustrate what the context of care is for these 25 clients--including the time of diagnosis, adjustment to regimens, daily living with a chronic condition, and relationships with health care providers. Their sense of history, current conflicts, and fears for the future are discussed as elements of the client's world.

At times during interviews, clients interpreted events differently than most providers would. Quotes exhibiting some of these differences have been included to emphasize that often clients do act and make decisions based on very different perspectives than providers usually hold.

The interviews which form the basis of this chapter were conducted with clients identified by public health and outpatient nurses. Clients were selected who: 1) had arthritis, COPD, diabetes or hypertension; 2) were currently in care and attempting to manage the chronic condition; and 3) were physically and emotionally able to participate in a 45-minute interview.

All clients were white, and from one of two Midwestern communities--a university town, or a small rural community quite distant from any major metropolitan area. Ages ranged from 23 to 73, with an average age of 54. The economic circumstances of individuals varied considerably: some were on medicaid, some had low-income jobs, some were retired, some had middle-ranged incomes, and two were university students.

TIME OF DIAGNOSIS

All of the clients interviewed were asked to describe the time of diagnosis--their own reactions, what had been most helpful during the visit, and what had been problematic. Clients told of experiencing many emotions at the time of diagnosis, including shock at learning they had a serious condition but also tremendous relief in learning what was wrong. Many had questioned their own sense that they were ill, particularly when families or providers did not take their concerns seriously. Following are quotes from four individuals:

> "I had been feeling bad all the time, I was aching all over
> and thought it was arthritis. I had a mixed reaction when
> I was told I had diabetes. First, it was a relief to know
> what was wrong, but also I was shocked. I didn't like it.
> My cousins, aunt, grandmother all had diabetes. My
> grandmother had gangrene and they wanted to amputate the
> foot. She wouldn't let them do it and she died. My aunt
> who had diabetes had her kidneys go bad and she died."

"I was really relieved to find out what it was. My stomach
felt empty all the time and I just felt strange. I was
relieved that it wasn't just in my head."

"It was a relief to find out that I wasn't imagining the
symptoms. Before that time I had headaches, but didn't
know what they were from."

"They put me in the hospital immediately and I had total
rest for 13 days. That was the best 13 days of that year.
Suddenly I was surrounded by people who knew what I had and
knew it wasn't just something in my head. I was so
relieved to finally find out what it was. Nothing is worse
than fear of the unknown."

For some, the relief of finding out what was wrong came later than for
others. Surprisingly, several of the clients interviewed found that their
concerns were not taken seriously, at least not at first. Thus, one man with
rheumatoid arthritis said:

"For five years I had pain in my shoulder, but I thought it
was from my job. The first physician just said I must have
a weak back. It kept on hurting, but they told me it
wasn't anything and there was nothing he could do. I'd
just have to handle it. It hurt so much sometimes at night
that I'd just cry. Finally, I got to a specialist and she
knew right away what it was."

A mother, worried about her four-year-old daughter, had the following
experience:

"I knew nothing about diabetes except that my brother, who
was a diabetic, always drank a lot of water. I was worried
that my daughter had diabetes because she was so tired and
drank so much water. All the doctor did was say, 'Don't
worry. Let's wait and see.' Well, I was really worried
about my daughter, and he just wouldn't listen. Finally,
after I kept insisting on tests he relented and found she
had 4+ urine. As soon as he found out, he wanted to
hospitalize her immediately. I said no, because I wanted a
chance to take her home and explain what the hospital was
like and what could be done. I didn't know what a
pediatric ward was like, and I wanted to know what kind of
bed she'd be put in and the number of kids she'd be with.
The doctor didn't care about any of that. All of a sudden,
when he finally took it seriously, he wanted to put her in
without any feeling of what it would do to her."

Another woman described the following scene:

"I told the doctor that I had trouble breathing and he took
some X-rays. After he looked at the X-rays he said my
lungs were fine. I said, 'Yes, but I can't breathe.' He

"said, 'Here, take these two prescriptions' without telling
me what they were for. I didn't want to go back after
that. My daughter convinced me when I couldn't breathe
that I had to see someone."

Several clients had vivid memories of their first interactions with providers,
and for some a substantial amount of disappointment or anger remains. A few
reported delaying going back for further diagnostic or treatment help as a
result of their early experience, and wondered if their health status might be
better now had they had been diagnosed earlier. It seems likely that these
memories influence client's subsequent perceptions and ability to work with
other providers.

Most clients said that clear explanations of the condition and tips on
self-management strategies were important during the first and early visits
following a diagnosis. Receiving handouts and newsletters seemed helpful.
The few family consultations that were reported were also quite significant as
these two examples suggest:

"Last year when I found out about the hypertension I
changed doctors and the new doctor wanted to meet my
husband. It really helped for him to do that. He talked
to both of us about why my blood pressure was important to
watch. He asked me why I thought it was up.... He
emphasized the importance of weight watching with my
husband. The doctor before was always too rushed.... My
new doctor takes time even when he has other patients."

"The doctor talked to me and my husband together. He
explained hypertension to us. It really helped that both
of us knew I wasn't imagining the symptoms."

The degree of provider sensitivity and efforts to explain the condition and
its management at the time of diagnosis were mentioned by several clients.
Some left the visit feeling they did not understand enough about the condition
to judge its seriousness. Others understood that the condition was serious,
but felt the doctor had been too cavalier in discussing it as these four
clients described:

"My doctor had been the family doctor for years and when he
gave me the diagnosis (of emphysema) he acted like it was
just another illness. Of course for me, it was a major
impact and change. But it almost seemed like he didn't
even take it seriously."

"I was hospitalized when I was losing weight. After five
days of tests, the doctor came in and said, 'Well, you've
got pernicious anemia and emphysema. We can control the
anemia, but with the emphysema, it's downhill all the way.'"

"The doctor didn't give any information to me or my
family. He wasn't very helpful. I wish he had said it was
serious and given more information about it."

>"When the doctor diagnosed my hypertension he scared me
>stiff. He said either take the pills and lose weight or
>I'd end up like my father, who had a stroke. He didn't
>explain what hypertension was."

To summarize, many of the clients' comments about the time of diagnosis
reflect a combination of relief and shock--relief to know what is wrong, but
fear or shock at the seriousness of the condition. In the midst of these
emotions, it appears that a provider's efforts to explain and answer questions
about the condition are extremely meaningful. Efforts to involve family and
to provide printed information seem further to aid a client's adjustment to
the condition. Similarly, lack of information, especially about the
seriousness of the condition, can be particularly significant. To some
clients who were dissatisfied with how things were handled at the time of
diagnosis, the lack of communication implied that the doctor did not take the
condition seriously. It may be that the providers were hesitant to discuss
the potentially upsetting prognosis. However, some clients indicated that
they might have managed their condition more closely had they been given more
information and a better indication of its seriousness from the beginning.

COPING WITH THE REGIMEN

Since self-management depends on the client's ability to understand and
follow the principles of the regimen, clients were asked how the original
regimens had worked out for them. Had there been any particular problems?
What in particular had helped them to follow the regimen? Responses varied
markedly. For some, there were virtually no problems, especially when the
regimen consisted solely of taking medication. For others, problems arose as
regimens became more complex or when their health status was not as good.
Sometimes the recommended regimen seemed unrealistic, because more activity or
energy was required than the client felt was currently possible.

>"My doctor told me I should try to get some exercise every
>day. He told me that each day I should increase it just a
>little bit more. He just doesn't understand that I can't
>breathe. I don't move anywhere unless I have to. He just
>doesn't understand what it's like...."

>"It's important for the doctor not to tell the patient he
>should do something when he really can't. You need to
>believe the patient and understand the signs of pain when
>they say they're in pain. Doctors need to take the patient
>more seriously. Even the first girl who took me in the
>wheelchair in the hospital understood more about pain than
>the doctor here in town. I just couldn't do most of what
>he told me to do."

These and other comments by clients suggest the frustration felt when the
client's physical limits aren't adequately understood and considered in
planning the recommended regimen. It may well be that providers were
encouraging clients to push themselves, and that the push was necessary to

achieve improvement; but from our interviews there seems to be a disparity between what the client and provider felt was realistic--and the disparity remained, or became greater, when not confronted.

A second concern voiced by some clients was that the regimens were very difficult to integrate into current family and job responsibilities. Some clients, while they wanted to follow the regimens, found it almost impossible to do so, given their current responsibilities. The regimens themselves presented a crisis: How could they follow the regimen and still maintain elements of their lifestyle which they and their families considered vital?

Clients deeply appreciated any practical tips for fitting the regimen into their lives:

> "The worst part at home was the mornings. I had to get my son off to school, my husband off to work; when the baby came I had to take care of her, and then besides we were trying to do urine tests on my daughter and give her shots in the morning. That was the low point of my life. It just wasn't humanly possible to do everything. Finally, out of desperation I called the public health nurses and asked if they could help. A nurse came and she had so many practical, innovative suggestions to fit with our family life. I was determined that we were going to have a good life, and I was determined that diabetes was not going to rule our life. I just can't tell you how much this one nurse helped us do this."

And yet not all advice is perceived by clients as practical.

> "The doctor told me I should rest more. When I work, I get more tired earlier. When I keep working it gets worse.... But I've got to work two jobs to make barely enough. If I can rest more, it'll help.... Walking and standing bothers me most, but I work in a factory where I'm on my feet most of the time."

> "They told me it was not curable and that I should plan to take aspirin and stop the aspirin when I was well. They also said I should rest 2-4 hours during the day and sleep 10-12 hours at night. That's impossible for someone with a 15-year-old. It's unrealistic. They should be more practical in how they deal with people."

The clients with diabetes identified urine testing and the subsequent decision making as a major challenge in their self-management efforts. Repeatedly people mentioned not being able to predict a schedule for eating and urine testing. The following was voiced by a 24-year-old woman who was diagnosed as diabetic when she was 13. She, more than any other of the individuals interviewed with diabetes, has tried to follow the regimen closely. She commented on the complexity which this introduces into her schedule, her relationships, and her own sense of control.

"I think the part that bothers me the most is the number of decisions that have to be made, and I'm a terrible decision maker. The kinds of things I have to do are planning where I will be after I leave the house.... If food is accessible, should I carry food, what kind of food I can carry (can I sit down and eat an orange or whatever), what kind of activity am I going to be doing. As far as the insulin dose in the morning, when is it going to peak? What am I going to be doing when it peaks? Am I going to have enough? And all that stuff that goes on before I leave the house while I am packing my bag in the morning; and those kinds of things now come naturally, but there were times when all I wanted to do was just get up and leave. Daily in the morning it's not bad, but when it gets to things like this past weekend when we were in Chicago... coordinating plans with other people, and you have to think--where will I be, and these people won't be ready to eat in two hours when I will have to eat... There's no way to get away from that. Well, you have to be conscious of it. You could overeat a meal so it will last for a while, but then you have to put up with feeling uncomfortable."

This particular young woman found herself weighing the benefits against the costs of trying to follow the regimen closely. Was it worth it to try to follow the regimen as closely as she was?

"When I started going to Jean for care was when I really started following all of this carefully. As I got the information, I really got into it. I often sit down and think about which way I was happier--before, when I wasn't trying to follow things as much, or afterwards, when I was. I wouldn't go back...but I would like to find a way to be a little less guilty about the whole thing, maybe I could know a little less, but I wouldn't go back. You do give something up, and I can understand why people say, 'Stop. I don't want anything more to do with it.'"

Another young woman, in college, described the problems that arose as she tried to maintain control in the midst of going to school:

"It's been a real challenge to keep myself regulated when I started school. Often I had classes at noon or from 4-7 right at the supper hour. I have to eat. It's a real problem; but I'll no sooner get adjusted to that, and I'll get my period and that throws it off. Or then exams will come along, and then there's Christmas break and the whole thing starts over again. I just get so frustrated with this whole thing, I just think I'll quit....You get things figured out and you hope things will just stay that way for a while. I just wanted to give up."

It seems that at times clients face a herculean task in trying to manage their condition. In the midst of such efforts clients welcome a partner who can be both nonjudgemental and helpful in problem solving; they want someone to help them deal with the inevitable barriers that arise.

"I have a doctor now who takes time and just listens and takes in what I say and works with it. He doesn't listen to it and try to ask, 'what is she really asking', or 'why here'. He just works with what I say. He tries to fit my diabetes care to my lifestyle rather than fit my lifestyle to my diabetes, because he knows I wouldn't do that anyway. He works on a problem until it is solved. He'll say, 'we'll keep working on it until we get it. We're not going to give up.' He always explains why he's doing something or why it is the way it is, how something (sickness) is affecting my diabetes, and what to watch for. He does a lot to help me problem solve; handle problems at home. I was just there, and he said to be sure if I had any problems to please let him know. I take that to mean that I don't have to wait until I'm dying, but I can call for lots of things, like if I'm having trouble regulating my diabetes or any little thing. I have a real sense of friendship and openness...just that he really cares, and that's very important to me."

"I was referred to Jean. I didn't want to go. It took me a year. I thought it was going to be the same old thing--she's still going to be a nurse, telling me what I should be doing--she's going to tell me how to do things and I'll say, 'sure, I'll do it', and then leave and not do it. When I went to see her, I gave the usual lines at first, and then the rest of the time I was really talking about it, and she was asking me what I wanted to do (and I wasn't afraid to say I didn't know). She was saying, 'OK, you want to lose weight, what are you willing to do for that? Are you willing to test with Clinitest?', and so on. I can't tell you what a feeling that was, just after a few months. I felt I was again controlling my disease, that I didn't ever have to lose consciousness again if I didn't want to."

Clients responded positively when providers appeared to accept problems with regimens as normal and were available to help when problems arose.

An additional need expressed was for basic information about why various aspects of the regimen were important. Just as clients had wanted the seriousness of the condition clearly acknowledged and explained, clients with more complex regimens also wanted the importance of specific aspects of the management plan explained. Some who had never understood their disease needed a fresh basic explanation:

"One of the most useful things she did was start from the beginning and talk about basics. She explained what the

disease process was and all of that....I probably heard
about it when I was first diagnosed, but that was nine
years ago and I just didn't remember much. I remember
being real strict for about three weeks, and after that
everything became a sort of mish-mash because I never got
any feedback on it. I probably did not want to ask anyone,
and nobody offered me the information....I didn't know if I
could trust her or not yet, but the approach was such that
I felt comfortable in saying that no, I didn't know what I
was doing and that's why I'm not doing it, it's because I
don't know why I'm urine testing."

The desire for information extended to clients who had fairly simple
regimens. For example, some wanted more information about possible side
effects of their drugs. They did not think that doctors were withholding this
information, but beleived doctors thought that clients already knew about the
side effects:

"At first when I had to take one of the medications a side
effect developed so that I could hardly walk; but the
doctor said I had to take them, so I did. Gradually I got
to ease off of that one. The doctor should have told me
what the side effects were because it really scared me. It
would save a lot of anxiety if doctors would tell us that
something unusual might happen....The doctor just takes for
granted that we know these things, but we don't."

"I noticed a depression from the anesthetic. I have a
nurse who explained that it was the anesthetic and not me.
The trouble with doctors is that they tend to forget that
the lay people don't know this."

Clients with hypertension often indicated that they wanted to know more
about a reduced sodium diet, having read and heard about it in the public
media.

Most said they wanted to reduce their salt but had difficulty doing this
without a diet developed specifically for them. It is not clear whether
clients had explicitly requested a diet, so many providers may have been
unaware of client interest.

"They didn't tell me anything about the diet; they just
gave me pills. I take my pills regularly, but I'm a
cheater about food. I love to eat, so I'd like to have a
diet for hypertension--on what to use for salt
substitutes. I try to read on my own now, but I'm not sure
what to use."

"The doctor didn't explain anything; he just prescribed the
pills. I take the pills faithfully, but it's hard to cut
out salt. I've never been given a diet to follow."

> "Diet is the hardest part of this. I didn't get much
> information about it, except from reading a Good
> Housekeeping article."

To summarize, clients are faced with major challenges in managing their
condition and providers can make a significant difference in how effective and
satisfying clients' self-management efforts are. The 25 clients interviewed
identified a need to have providers consider their physical limitations as
well as their social and work responsibilities when designing and negotiating
the self-management scheme. Clients also expressed the need for information
about the condition and the regimen, and for problem-solving help with the
regimen as questions arose. At least some of the clients described their
relationships with providers as being very supportive, and yet task-focused.
When clients perceived their providers as open and nonjudgemental, it seemed
they were more likely to raise questions about management problems. Part of
the challenge for providers is to establish the foundation on which such
openness can be built. Another part of the challenge is to judge how much and
what kind of information will be useful for each client across a series of
visits.

COPING WITH THE CONDITION

The clients we interviewed wanted to lead normal, active lives. Fitting a
regimen into their lives often challenged this goal, particularly when
problems associated with the condition had already caused disruptions. When
self-management is viewed from this perspective, it is easier to see why the
added burden of the regimen might be resented: as if the condition itself were
not enough, now the client has to cope with a regimen, too. To clarify just
how much the condition alone changes a client's life, we asked clients what
types of changes, if any, they had made after the diagnosis.

For people with COPD, the loss of breathing ability seemed to affect their
entire pattern of activity. Roles within the family changed, personal sources
of pride were challenged, and social contacts diminished as the ability to
breath decreased. The general tone in these interviews was one of loss.

> "Since getting ill I haven't encouraged any out-of-town
> guests who used to come for visits. That was something we
> used to do a lot and really looked forward to. But what's
> the point now? You say one sentence, and that's it. A
> conversation is impossible now."

Another person talked about the loss of her independence and
mobility:

> "Driving the car is impossible. I just don't feel secure
> enough to do that. I don't even think that I could open
> the doors or the garage door. I'm much more dependent than
> I ever was. I have family and friends who come by but I
> don't go out at all like I used to."

A third individual talked about personal loss in terms of objects and links to family members now dead:

> "I had to get rid of house plants; I couldn't take care of them. And then I moved from my second-floor apartment to the first floor because I couldn't walk up the steps. And then I had to get rid of all my feather pillows and quilts that my mother had given me. They were beautiful, and some of the last things I had from her."

Pride and the desire to lead a normal life, particularly with family, appears to be one of the hardest challenges for clients to resolve:

> "I have worked and done the housework besides, and tended to downplay the pain the whole time. The pain was there, but it wasn't so bad that I couldn't keep going. As a result, I didn't take care of myself. I have had nine surgical operations because of it.... The thing that is hardest now is to swallow my pride and ask for help. I resent the fact that I have to ask for help--who am I punishing? I'm too proud to let them help...."

> "Your pride is affected. My wife can do everything in about one third the time that I can do it, but I'm from the old school and so that's not something I can live with easily."

Several clients indicated that they did not want to be viewed as different from other people, and at times took considerable risks with their health to maintain the social image of being normal:

> "A few months ago I had a hypoglycemic reaction at work and I was very hesitant to tell anyone what was happening. I felt that they would act like it was a problem and that I couldn't handle it."

> "The other day when I was mowing my lawn I took a little stool out to sit on for when I can't breathe. When people drove by they probably thought I was pretty strange. I hate doing that."

> "The big thing for me was I didn't care if people knew I had diabetes, but I didn't want to be different from anyone else. So I'd hide whenever I needed snacks, or sometimes I'd just skip them."

Thus, it seems that in addition to coping with considerable disruption in their lives, directly attributable to the medical condition, several clients we interviewed also contended with fears of being viewed as different. They put considerable thought and effort into maintaining an image of being normal in the family, at work, and in public among strangers and friends. Having people know their diagnosis was less a problem than needing to act differently than others in order to manage the condition.

Another dimension of client concerns identified through our interviews was fear of complications associated with the chronic condition. All clients were asked whether they had any major fears about their condition. The response indicated that they had done substantial thinking about complications and disabilities. Although the nature of the fears varied, especially between clients with different chronic conditions, each responded with clearly identified, personally devastating outcomes. Following are some of the examples, grouped by the different chronic conditions.

Clients with arthritis mentioned fears such as these two:

"My biggest fear is becoming deformed. I just don't want that to happen. I guess another big thing I'm really frightened about is losing my physician. She's the first one who has understood what was happening and has given me medications that could help with the pain. She may leave, and I don't know what I'll do then. It took so long to find her and nobody else believed me when I said how much pain I was in...or at least they didn't know what to do to help. I used to have so much pain that I had to cry, and still the doctor would say there was nothing anyone could do."

"I'm most afraid of what's going to happen down the road. They can only do so much surgery. I'm afraid I'll lose the use of my hands and feet. I'm not as concerned about the pain. I've lived with that most of my life."

While fears of deformity and lack of mobility seemed uppermost to clients with arthritis, those with COPD worried about suffocation:

"I get to feeling so panicky when I'm short of breath. It feels like you are on a constant treadmill. I'm terrified of the time I won't be able to breathe at all."

"It's like a constant struggle for breath...sort of like when I almost drowned when I was six years old. The food just gushed out of my nose and mouth and I couldn't breathe. That's what it's like for me now often. My biggest fear is that I'm finally going to suffocate. You know you just can't get those satisfying breaths anymore. Occasionally I can get them, but I'd do anything to be able to get those satisfying breaths."

Clients with insulin-dependent diabetes expressed fears about losing consciousness and the end-stage complications which can occur:

"Well, my biggest fear is going blind. But I'm also afraid of passing out."

"I don't feel like I have any escape. I know that sometime down the road the complications are going to hit me, just like they've hit my friend. She's 32 or 33 and so it

really made an impact. She has every complication in the
book. She's had to have some amputations, she's going
blind, and her kidneys are just about shot....I've had
diabetes from 15 years, and I just keep thinking...'It's
just a matter of waiting; I'm sure they're going to come.'"

The clients with hypertension consistently identified stroke as their most
prominent concern:

"I think hypertension is a lot like cancer. You can't
control the causes or recognize it until it's way too
late. My biggest fear is a massive stroke."

"My biggest fear is a stroke. I would live on and wouldn't
be able to function normally."

One interview was particularly interesting in that when the client was
asked about possible fears, his wife started to respond, but the client
interrupted and said, "No, that's not right." He explained that blindness was
his biggest fear; this was a revelation to his wife. For him and probably for
others, it was difficult to discuss fears even with close family or friends.
A provider may need to encourage clients to express their concerns.

From the way in which clients responded when asked about their major
fears, it seemed that a fair amount of emotional energy had gone into thinking
about the complications which would be most devastating for the individual.
They also had developed a variety of ways to cope with these fears. One
client started meeting with a group of peers. She indicated that the group
helped her discuss her fears about complications:

"At one point I joined a group with other women who had
insulin-dependent diabetes. It was great to find out that
other people were having the same troubles, and that there
were other people that were feeling as overwhelmed with the
guilt and monitoring. I looked to the group for a feeling
of relief by being able to share all of this. We talked a
lot about how we felt when we cheated--meaning when we ate
a lot--and I think that a lot of it just centered around
that and feeling guilty about it.... A lot of us mentioned
how our minds became little computers, and every time we
looked at food you always broke it down into exchanges--and
how irritating that gets; and about trying to decide that
you might want to be more relaxed and enjoy yourself,
trying to do that, but at the same time, in the back of
your head, you are still thinking about long-term
complications. When we were eating or drinking, whatever,
we were still thinking (about complications).... One girl
was talking about how she can just feel her high blood
sugar going through her veins and wrecking her, and it's
hard."

Interviews with clients who have hypertension suggested another mechanism by which clients may cope with their fears. These people represented a fairly unusual group in that their regimens and symptoms, on the surface at least, seemed to disrupt their lives somewhat less than for other clients interviewed. Their fears of stroke, however, seemed just as anxiety producing. Many were aware of family and friends who had suffered strokes as a result of hypertension. Out of their own and others' experience most had developed ideas about the cause of their hypertension and what was necessary to control or "cure" it. Most attributed their elevated blood pressure to stress, rather than to any inherent physical predisposition. An important means of coping with the condition, therefore, in addition to taking medications, was to manage stress better:

>"My mother, sister, and husband all have had hypertension. My husband had a stroke from it and now I'm the sole breadwinner. My mother was moody, withdrawn, she cried a lot. There were no pills. In those days you didn't take pills for stress. It used to be called 'nerves' but now it's called stress.... I think that the stress from my husband's stroke caused my hypertension. I also started a new job and lifestyle. I'm pretty sure I know when my blood pressure is going up. I have headaches in the front of my head, and I get red from the neck up.... Pressure from my job creates more stress and anger and that causes it to go up.... The best thing for me to do to prevent it from going up is just to leave the situation. I try to get away. Get a change of environment. I try to forget it and do something like get my hair done. I try to relax more at home. I take time to get away. The children are gone so that helps."

>"I tell myself that it's mind over matter, not to get upset when I feel my blood pressure is up. I just try to slow down and relax, take time out. I do needlework. When I run out of things to do I get too nervous. It makes me imagine what's wrong when I get nervous.... The biggest change is that I try to use mind over matter. Not to let things get me upset. I try not to overtax my body. I try to just sit and turn off my mind. I feel that my attitude has changed. Before, I used to fly off the handle, but now I feel less angry."

>"My father's stroke raised my blood pressure and made me more nervous.... I can feel when my blood pressure goes up. I get headaches, flushed in the face, and dizzy. I go to the doctor and he changes my pills then.... It changes with what's happening to me emotionally. When I'm under stress it goes up. If I rest during a crisis it seems like my blood pressure goes down."

>"I know when it's going up. I get nervous and jittery. It usually happens when I get worried about something. Worry always makes it worse.... What I do then is try to relax.... I sew or do something with my hands."

As these quotes suggest, a large number of the clients interviewed had perceptions not entirely consistent with the medical model of hypertension. Although the literature generally describes hypertension as symptomless, most clients felt that they could tell quite clearly when their blood pressure was elevated, and often described very similar symptoms: flushed face, headache, jitters, dizziness. Similar findings are reported in a major study by Meyer (1980). This is an example of a discrepancy between client and provider perspectives that can lead to less open communication between client and provider and can lead to major disagreement about self-management regimens. From the client's perspective, causes and symptoms of stress coupled with stress-management techniques may have seemed very important. However, since no clients reported having received information on stress, it appears that sources, symptoms, and management of stress were less important to providers.

RECOMMENDATIONS FOR PRACTICE

As a final question, all of the clients interviewed were asked if they had any recommendations for health providers, based on their own experience as clients. Their responses, brief but clear, help communicate their perspective of what the client-provider partnership should be. These concerns can be grouped under three general headings: information, communication, and resources.

Information

The clients interviewed indicated that they need and want to know more fully about their chronic condition: the simple tricks and coping mechanisms for the day-to-day difficulties of living with their condition, the basic description of the condition and its treatment, and a full understanding of possible risks and complications.

> "Clients like me should be able to learn how to breathe correctly. I didn't realize it was possible until the group I joined. I suppose the doctors assume that you know about that, but you don't!"

> "It's really helpful when they give you recipes and cookbooks for diabetes. We need to learn as much as we can about the disease and what to do for it."

> "I was only vaguely aware of complications when I was first diagnosed. For all I knew, it could have been tough skin in not getting the needle in. Honestly, I saw Buddy Epson on TV and he said that diabetes was the leading cause of blindness in the country and that was the first time that I realized the severity of the complication. I think providers should bring this up so that people aren't hit suddenly with a complication who have never had the information and who feel that they never had a chance to do something about it."

Providers can help by not assuming the client already knows as much as he or she wants to know. Discussion about complications appeared to be as important to some clients as hints for daily living were to others. The provider is a unique resource to the client in preventing fears and mistakes based on ignorance.

"Doctors should tell patients what to expect with their emphysema. Some people might want to be pollyanna-ish. But I really want to know the truth. Just because you do all the things you should and hope for the best doesn't mean it's going to turn out all right."

Communication

As with most aspects of the client-provider relationship, information does not stand alone. It is communicated in a particular way, and clients' comments suggested that they were sensitive to how as well as what was communicated. Interviewed clients wanted follow-up and discussion of the decisions that are made, the regimen chosen, and the tests and measures of their condition.

"When doctors ask you to do something like urine testing they should follow up on it and discuss it at each visit instead of just glancing at the card. My doctor used to just look at the values and sometimes he'd say, 'You should probably be doing better.' It would have been a lot more helpful if he had helped me try to find the reason why I was running those 4+'s at night. It was hard to know if I should take it seriously if he didn't."

They wanted the realities of their own lives taken into consideration:

"It's really helpful to have the doctor talk with you and your husband together. It helped him to understand a lot of what I was going through...."

"Doctors shouldn't simply tell patients what they're supposed to do. They should find out what the patient is going to do and then work with that. Help them make the choices as safely as possible, but have the patients make the choices and have some sense of control."

"Doctors should be very practical in the suggestions they make for patients. If it's not realistic, patients aren't going to do it."

They wanted to be listened to, and they wanted to feel free to ask little questions, to call at the beginning of a concern and not only when there is a full crisis.

"They should spend enough time that patients can ask questions without feeling so rushed."

"I want someone who will listen carefully to what I say and take it as I say it, not try to make something different out of it."

"I think that patients should be encouraged to call when
they have questions. Sometimes you feel like it's only
okay to call or see someone if it's something serious. But
if you could feel comfortable asking for information or
help earlier it might not have to get serious."

Sometimes the provider will need to listen for the unexpressed
request, or even for denial. How often is a wishful bit of hope,
like this statement spoken by a man with severe emphysema, expressed
in a clinical setting?

"I wish the doctors could show me what my lungs look like
since I stopped smoking last year. It was so hard to do
that I'd just like to know. Maybe they're all nice and
healthy pink now."

Communication is not only verbal:

"Doctors should be gentle when they touch you."

Resources

Interviewed clients indicated they want and need the full use of a provider's
resources, including their ability to make appropriate referrals, and to offer
basic resources of time and support.

It may be that a provider is unable to respond to a client's need;
referrals were viewed as just as appropriate then.

"I want someone who is assertive in using resources on my
behalf--not someone who would be defensive about making
referrals or having consultations."

"Doctors should be straightforward. If they know how to
care for a problem they should do it. If not, they
shouldn't monkey with it. The doctor should send the
patient to a specialist."

Time is a resource essential to communication and information, but valuable
enough by any standards to be considered separately. Noted above is the
importance to these clients of time to ask questions, time to be heard.
Clients also need time for problem-solving and time to talk, for talking can
be in itself a release, needed before other elements in the overall care can
happen:

"I want a person who I can bounce my concerns off of and
who will listen and then help me to do something about my
concern. I need the person to help me problem solve what
the next step should be."

"It's really important to understand that arthritis is
painful and that people with arthritis have to talk about
the pain more than others because it is so painful. People
should understand that we're not just complaining."

And one last vital resource (not without its time and communication aspects) is commitment. The person with a chronic condition has long-term, demanding needs for care:

> "I want someone who will stick with a problem until we make progress with it."

> "If a patient is suffering severe problems or complications it's important not to abandon him. The most important thing would be to tell the person that you'd be there no matter what happened. After that, I think that at that stage, one of the big issues might be just talking. A person may feel guilt or anger. I would think that it would be universal, that you would think back over every time you ate, and every time you didn't do your testing and every time you did anything wrong. I think being able to talk about these things with a health care person would be good--someone who would then say that it's in the past. We have to deal with what is happening to you now. I think the major issue with chronic illness is that there are times when there is nothing else that you can do except sit and listen. And actually that's a lot."

The last quote suggests that at times the provider's primary contribution may be his or her full attention, and a commitment not to sever the client-provider relationship. If, indeed, the earlier phases of the provider-client relationship have been marked by a growing trust and openness, one can imagine what a gift it would be to have this relationship continue during the client's final efforts to grapple with the reality of complications.

Unfortunately, continuity of provider contact is often disrupted when severe complications and hospitalization occur, which underscores the need to encourage clients to become as independent as possible in asking for and getting what they need. The following chapter offers suggestions for how providers can promote client independence through active involvement during the client visit.

CHAPTER 3
DEVISING AND REVISING THE REGIMEN

As the preceding chapter suggests, it is much easier to help clients help themselves when the context of their lives is understood--what losses they have experienced due to the condition, what degree of adjustment has been necessary, and who has been helpful in this effort. Although initially more time may be spent on formal assessment, many of these issues can be raised only through informal and ongoing conversations across several visits. When the client is involved actively as a partner during the visit, aspects of his or her life can be identified informally as they become relevant to the planning and problem solving at hand.

To aid the process of involving clients actively during visits, this chapter focuses on the 1:1 interaction between client and provider. Concrete suggestions for assessment, communication process, and problem solving will be described. The goal is to involve clients actively in each visit in order to promote their self-management.

It is important to acknowledge that clients vary in their ability and willingness to participate in decision making and self-management. Some, particularly those who are newly diagnosed, or in crisis, may not be able to enter into a partnership for a while. Others may not be ready to step out of a familiar, more traditional relationship. A client in crisis (or one who resists active participation) may seem somewhat disoriented, have difficulty understanding new information, lose eye contact frequently, or give only vague responses. At such times only minimal education should be attempted, with the primary focus on immediate needs. The provider may need to be more directive and to model problem solving rather than expect the client to join actively. A follow-up appointment can be scheduled fairly soon and involvement of family or other resources, such as visiting nurses, might be considered. If enough time is available to reach closure, it may also help to encourage the client to talk about his or her concerns.

When clients who have experienced traditional provider-client relationships are reluctant to change, the provider may need to be more of a traditional authority figure. Nonetheless, over time, significant opportunities for client input into planning various parts of the regimen will arise, so it is important not to take the responsibility for decision making out of the client's hand unnecessarily. The client can be encouraged to make such decisions as "where to put my pills so that I'll remember to take them." In the process, small steps toward a larger self-management role may be made. Ultimately, however, the extent to which a client is actively involved in decisions and care depends to a great extent on the client.

DEVISING THE CONSENSUAL REGIMEN

The term consensual regimen refers to a regimen devised through consensus, or mutual negotiation between the client and provider (Fink, 1976). In his excellent essay, Fink points out several assumptions upon which the consensual regimen is based: 1) There is no such thing as a standard regimen for a standard client; every regimen is in some sense a negotiated one, and each client, with his illness, presents a new combination of circumstances to which the regimen must be adapted. 2) Health decisions and behavior are carried out in the context of the total life setting. Current life priorities, family, and social stress affect the management of health and illness, and the provider must therefore gather such information about the client and his or her family life. 3) The universe of health problems of a particular individual is always changing and at times requires the client to be self-sufficient in solving some of these health problems.

In Fink's model, clients play an active role in the development of their own regimens; this assures that client priorities, lifestyle, and resources are considered. Fink (1976) and other authors of adherence literature (Becker and Maiman, 1980; Haynes, 1979; 1980; Meyer, 1980; Sackett, 1976; Steckel, 1981) suggest that the following concerns must be addressed as client and provider develop the regimen:

. What is the client's priority and source of motivation?

. What level of self-management is realistic for the client at this point?

. How can the regimen best be tailored to client activities, both for convenience and to remind clients to take medications?

. How does the proposed self-management task mesh with the client's own ideas or models of the condition and its management?

. Would the client like to involve anyone to support and encourage his or her self-management?

. Is the self-management task defined concretely and clearly in behavioral terms?

In this chapter each of these questions is discussed briefly. Table 3 summarizes assessment and provides examples of how the information can be gathered.

Client Priorities

As Korsch and Negrete (1972) demonstrated in their study of 800 client visits, the majority of clients come to an appointment with a clear agenda, and a significant proportion leave without discussing their primary concern. Korsch and Negrete found that adherence was lowest among clients who felt that the provider had not dealt with the client's concern. One implication from this research is that it is particularly important to identify what the client wants help with, and to design regimens which respond to the client's major concern, as well as the provider's. For example, a client with arthritis may be preoccupied with pain. If the client feels the regimen helps to reduce the pain, the likelihood of adherence is heightened. Often the provider can explain to the client how the recommended regimen will help reduce pain. The important thing is to identify and address the client's priority issues immediately or, if time is a problem, make an appointment to do so.

A client with diabetes interviewed for this book provides one example. At her first visit with a new provider, this client presented a history of nonadherence, with frequent trips to the emergency room--most recently because she had been dieting without adequately regulating her diabetes. As the provider talked with the client, she tried to identify what goal the client most wanted to work toward at this point. At first the client said that she didn't know; however, after a few minutes she said that losing weight was her priority. Rather than discourage this, the provider responded positively and asked what the client was willing to do in order to lose weight. Was she willing to test with Clinitest? Regulate her diet? Come in every two weeks? If yes, she would help the client set up a diet to lose weight. Motivated primarily by her concern about being overweight, the client entered into the joint process of planning a regimen by which she could both lose weight and regulate her diabetes.

Level of Self-Management

One of the most critical steps in regimen planning is judging accurately what level of self-management the client wants and is able to assume. This judgement is based in part on the socio-emotional context of the client's life. Are there other stressors, such as family problems or job loss? How much energy does the client exhibit? How much of the client's energy is tied up in adjusting to a sense of lost health or diminished quality of life?

Does the client's language and behavior suggest hopelessness, as opposed to a sense of internal control (Genther, 1981)? Further examples of factors affecting client readiness for self-management are given in Table 3.

When assessment suggests that the client has a limited attention span, low interest, and low energy for self-management, the regimen should be kept as simple as possible. The adherence research suggests that generally it is more difficult for people to follow complex regimens than it is to follow fairly simple ones (Sackett, 1976). The contracting literature, furthermore, suggests that client success is the key to shaping client behaviors. Regimens should focus only on tasks that the client believes he or she can perform successfully (Steckel, 1977). Unfortunately, a client's perceptions may differ from a provider's on what is a "do-able" task. A doctor may tell the client with COPD that she should exercise daily, building each day on the amount of exercise done the day before; but the client may feel that she has barely enough energy and breath to do her minimum tasks. Thus, in this example, the doctor's advice would have, if anything, a demoralizing effect.

TABLE 3. ASSESSMENT

Information Sought	Examples of provider questions or observations
I. CLIENT PRIORITIES	
A. <u>Key client concerns and expectations for visit</u>	"What would you most like to have us cover today?" "Is there anything you're concerned about right now?" "How have things been going? Any questions come up?" [At end of visit:] "Is there anything else we should cover today? Is there something you'd like me to look into [or think about] for next time?"
B. <u>Client fears</u>	"Are there any [worst] fears that you have about_____?" "You mentioned that your mother had a stroke. Does this worry you at all?"
II. CLIENT SELF-MANAGEMENT LEVEL	
A. <u>Client readiness</u>	-- Prior pattern of seeking information -- Current pattern of monitoring condition -- Energy level -- Pattern of responding to crises (actively, passively) -- Pattern of language (exhibiting internal vs. external control)
B. <u>Client ability to concentrate and to integrate new information</u>	-- Loss of eye contact -- Vague responses -- Frequent confusion -- Directing provider to others (e.g., "I think my wife knows about that.")
C. <u>Sense of loss</u>	"What has changed most in your life since you found you have_____?"
D. <u>Current stressors</u>	"What other stresses are you or your family under right now?"
E. <u>Client need for self-management</u>	-- Living alone -- Single head of household -- Complex lifestyle precludes frequent health care visits -- Pride or fear of dependence -- Distrust of medical setting/provider -- Distance from clinic

TABLE 3. ASSESSMENT (continued)

Information Sought	Examples of provider questions or observations
III. TAILORING THE REGIMEN	
A. <u>Lifestyle</u>	"Describe a typical day. When do you get up, eat your meals?" "What do you do for fun?" "When during the week are you most likely to get together with other people?" "For what things are you likely to go out of the house?" "What is a typical day of work like?"
B. <u>Sense of loss</u>	"How has your life changed since having _____?" "What has been important to keep the same?"
C. <u>Client prior experience with other regimens</u>	"People often say they have trouble with their medications, remembering them, or sometimes trouble with side effects. Was this true for you then, at all? Did you discover any special way of keeping track?" "How often did you find you took your pills -- some of the time, most of the time, not too often? What tended to interfere? What helped you to remember?" "Did you discover any special way of keeping track?" "Have you tried to lose weight before? What happened then?" "What seemed to help you the most to stay on your diet? What got in the way? What was the hardest about staying on? Is there anything you'd do differently this time?
IV. THE CLIENT'S MODEL	
A. <u>Client model of the condition and its management</u>	"When did you first notice _____?" "What do you think caused it?" "Are there times it gets worse or better? How do you tell?" "Does anything seem to make it better or worse?"
B. <u>Prior contact with others who had condition</u>	"Have you known anyone else who had _____? What happened with them? How were they treated?

TABLE 3. ASSESSMENT (continued)

Information Sought	Examples of provider questions or observations
C. Client knowledge, misperceptions	"How have you learned about _____? What did [the source] say about it?" "It helps to find out what you already know, so I can focus our time on what you don't know. To start with, is there anything you particularly want to know? What about [urine testing]? In how much detail was that covered? Tell me about your medication. When do you take it? What does it do? How do you store it?"
D. Prior experience with health care system	"Tell me about the time of diagnosis. What was that like?"

V. SOCIAL SUPPORT

A. Current support system: who is most important	[Often provided in medical history.] "You mentioned that you live alone now with your wife. Have you discussed your _____ with her? How has she taken it? Would it be helpful if she came to the next visit and we explained what's going on and how she can help?" "Who has been most helpful since you found out you have _____?" "Is there anyone who has been especially helpful to you in the past?" "What kind of help is hard for you to ask for?" "What help are your famiy and friends especially good at giving? What else do you still need?"

It is difficult to know at times how to enhance clients' perceptions of their own capacities. If the client's condition requires a more complex regimen, a variety of strategies discussed in detail in subsequent chapters can be used. The provider may have to explore several strategies, such as a contracting or family involvement, with clients whose motivation and energy for self-management are low.

Low energy for self-management is not always the problem and simplicity of regimen is not always the best answer. Another aspect to consider in deciding "how much--how fast--how complex a regimen" goes back to what the client wants to learn and what the client's key concerns are. One client with hypertension may want to learn about a salt-free diet right away, although providers frequently tend to introduce medications alone at first. Another client with hypertension may be extremely interested in learning to take her own blood pressure. A third client may have so much pain from her arthritis that she is willing to undertake a fairly complex medication schedule to control pain. While it is important to avoid overloading the client with a complex self-management regimen, the negotiation process between client and provider may well result in a very different combination of tasks than the provider would have selected, had he or she been focusing solely on simplicity of regimen.

Tailoring the Regimen

As Mullen (1980) has noted, clients with a chronic condition are constantly trying to balance quality of life issues against the need to follow regimens which can slow or prevent the degenerative effects of the condition. Clients interviewed for this book expressed how frustrating this can be. Some clients choose to ignore regimens completely, rather than alter patterns in their lives. Thus, efforts are well spent in tailoring the regimen to the client's particular daily schedule of activities and priorities.

The simplest example of tailoring a regimen can be seen in planning a medication schedule. The goal is to arrive at a medication schedule that will be most convenient and easy for the client to follow (Fink, 1976). Such a schedule is not intrusive, helps to minimize the inconvenience of side effects and can be scheduled around regular habits.

The provider cannot achieve the goal without understanding what the client's day (and night) look like, and what activities are particularly significant and/or habitual within the schedule. With this information, specific cues for taking the medication can be identified. For example, a man's medications can be stored where he is likely to be when they are needed, e.g., by his razor in the bathroom. Habitual activities, such as meals or bedtime, can act as cues even when not tied to a specific place.

Zifferblatt and Curry (1977) point out that providers may wish to encourage some clients to write down what they were doing when they either took or forgot their medication (the occasion, people present, behavior, thoughts, what happens afterwards). They encourage clients to pretend they are looking at a motion picture of themselves around medication-taking time and simply record what they can see. As clients observe and record this information, they become more aware of the events that influence their medication taking. A sample record, completed by a client, appears in Figure 1.

Another aspect of tailoring a regimen is trying to preserve what the client perceives to be special in his or her schedule or habits. Given that clients often have to adjust to major losses resulting from the condition, it is useful to problem-solve ways to minimize further losses caused by the regimen itself. Clients therefore need to identify current habits and activities which help make life worth living. Whether these events occur daily or yearly, anything that provides particular pleasure--visiting with grandchildren, going out weekly with the guys, eating a particular food, attending church bazaars--should be incorporated into the proposed regimen whenever possible. The proposed regimen will then allow for the things that contribute most to the client's quality of life. The regimen may not always appear to permit this flexibility, but good problem-solving usually results in a compromise. For example, a client with hypertension noted that one of the big joys in her life was having her grandchildren over each Monday evening. The medication prescribed could have caused some undesirable side effects during this time, so the medication schedule was adjusted to minimize the likelihood that her time with her grandchildren would be spoiled.

Many clients have past experiences and information that is extremely useful for anticipating potential problems or strategies with the regimen. To identify patterns in client behavior, ask questions in as nonjudgemental a way as possible. The following questions often yield useful information:

> "Did anything tend to get in the way of your using the splints? Tell me what that was like."

> "How often were you able to do your breathing exercises? Never? Some of the time? Most of the time? Why do you think that was?"

> "Some people say they have trouble with their medications-- either remembering them or with side effects. Did this happen with you also? What happened?"

Asking clients about any problems they might have had reinforces the message that the provider and client can adjust the regimen based on the client's needs and experience with it.

Whether regimens involves exercise, stress management, diet changes, joint protection, breathing exercises, or postural drainage, the more precisely clients can identify the events that precede or follow the proposed self-management tasks, the easier it will be to tailor the regimen to the client's needs. Thus, the provider may wish to suggest that the client begin systematically to observe events preceding and following the self-management tasks as scheduled. In subsequent visits the client and provider can then problem-solve ways to increase the ease of carrying out the regimen or can modify expectations for the regimen itself. The more the regimen can be adapted to the client's circumstances, the more likely it is to be followed.

Medication-Taking Record

	Time	Occasion	People	Behavior	Thoughts	What Happens After
Day 1						
Day 2						
Day 3						

Sample Medication-Taking Record

	Time	Occasion	People	Behavior	Thoughts	What Happens After
Day 1	9:00 A.M.	breakfast orange juice	Helen	take medication	glad I remembered hope it decreases my appetite	ate breakfast nothing special
	9:00 P.M.	TV	Helen			
Day 2	9:40 A.M.	reminded by Helen as I was leaving for work		take medication	I don't care if I remember this will make me drowsy	nothing special went to work
	9:30 P.M.	reading a book	Helen		this is too difficult	nothing went to bed
Day 3	8:30 A.M.	brushing teeth reminded by Helen		take medication	Helen is a nag makes me too sleepy	had breakfast
	10.00 P.M.	getting into bed	Helen		can't seem to remember	went to bed

Develop your own system of codes, but make sure you put it on the back of the record so you don't forget it and can understand your recording.

FIGURE 1. SAMPLE OF MEDICATION-TAKING RECORD AND A RECORD COMPLETED BY A CLIENT

Reprinted, from Medciation Compliance: A Behavioral Approach, with permission, from Charles B. Slack, Inc., 1981.

Identifying the Client's Ideas About the Condition

The client's own ideas about the condition and its management also are important to assess (Meyer, 1980; Leventhal and others, 1980). An assumption underlying Meyer and Leventhal's work is that people approach illness just as they do other crises and problems in their lives. They use prior personal impressions and knowledge of others' experiences to understand the problem at hand. They try to observe what seems to improve or worsen symptoms and then formulate a "picture," or model, of the chronic condition and its treatment.

Quotes in Chapter 1 from several people interviewed for this book suggest the same pattern or model. Clients with hypertension tended to attribute their condition to a particular cause (e.g., stress). They identified specific symptoms (e.g., headaches) they felt were associated with elevated blood pressure. They also described interventions (e.g., stress management) which they thought reduced their blood pressure.

The danger is that the client's picture of the disease may be inconsistent with the provider's model. Thus, the provider needs to identify what assumptions the client has about the condition and its treatment that could influence commitment to a regimen. Examples of the kinds of questions to ask are provided in Table 3.

If, as Meyer suggests, some clients also tend to view their chronic condition as episodic or acute, these clients may discontinue treatment when symptoms disappear (e.g. when headaches stop). Thus a regimen calling for medications even when symptoms are absent might conflict with the client's understanding of the condition and would therefore be less likely to be implemented. One approach to this problem is to help the client develop a more accurate model of his or her condition. For example, self-blood pressure monitoring is one option for the client with hypertension. The client would record blood pressure levels at regular intervals, regardless of the presence or absence of symptoms. The measures become feedback on the accuracy of using symptoms to infer whether blood pressure is elevated. Two things are accomplished by this type of intervention. First, the client's interest in monitoring his or her symptoms and blood pressure is reinforced rather than denied. Second, it is likely that the client would learn that blood pressure can be elevated even when symptoms are absent and thus that medication is needed on a continuous basis.

Social Support

A number of adherence reviews cite social support as an important resource to self-management efforts by clients (Becker, 1980; Dunbar et al., 1979; Hogue, 1979; Haynes, 1976). Green et al. (1975) found that 70% of clients studied with hypertension reported a need for greater family support and knowledge with respect to the client's condition. Many clients apparently would like to see more family involvement.

In the process of devising the regimen, there is usually an opportunity to ask the client whether he or she wants a family member or significant other involved in some way. If the answer is affirmative, there are a number of strategies available, as described in Chapter 5. At minimum a family member or friend can attend a client visit to learn more about the client's condition and management. In addition, if the client wishes, the person can provide support by encouraging the client's efforts, witnessing any behavioral contracts, and helping to facilitate management (joint meal-planning, providing special incentives to help motivate the client). The goal of family involvement is to develop an ally who can help reduce roadblocks, increase ease of management, and provide positive feedback for successes.

A variety of strategies can help generate social support for clients with chronic conditions who are older and living alone. Sometimes a client can identify a significant other with whom she or he has meaningful contact (a sibling, neighbor, church member). Such a person might provide support through telephone contact, or by witnessing a behavioral contract which the client might develop with the provider. At other times, a client may need to be encouraged to join a support group for individuals with the same chronic condition. Through the group, the client may meet others who can continue to play a support role after the group sessions end. Depending on the provider's resources, card or telephone contact with the client may be a third strategy to consider.

Clear Definition of Tasks

The client needs to understand how to follow the regimen before leaving a visit or a hospitalization. While this may seem so obvious as to be trite, research suggests that a surprising number of clients often do not follow regimens because they are confused (Boyd, 1974; Svarstad, 1976). Boyd found that over 60% of the clients in their study misunderstood the physician's verbal instructions about the method for taking medication. More than half of the clients studied by Svarstad (1976) made at least one error in describing the physician's expectations approximately one week after the clinic visit. At least part of this confusion results from imprecise or overly brief instructions (Stone, 1979). For example, "take with meals" was interpreted by clients intending to adhere to instructions as meaning to take medications as much as an hour before or after the meal. Work by Hulka (1979) indicates that as the number of medications to be taken increase, the probability of errors in medication adherence also increases. The need for clear instructions is all the more necessary when multiple medications or tasks are required.

One benefit of jointly negotiating a regimen with the client is that the process of tailoring will help to define the client's tasks in concrete terms. To confirm that tasks are clearly defined, it is useful to write them down and compare them with the client's expectations. The tasks should be clear enough that they can be written in the form of a contract, regardless of whether a contract is going to be used. A natural opportunity to do this can occur if the provider records the plan in the client's file to serve as a follow-up reminder for the next visit.

MONITORING AND REVISING REGIMENS

Monitoring the client's conformity to the regimen during later visits is at least as important as originally devising the regimen. Monitoring provides the opportunity for a variety of functions to occur in a natural way. First, it allows the provider to indicate indirectly but clearly that the regimen is important for management of the condition. There is some evidence from our client interviews (presented in Chapter 1) that when a provider did not monitor regimens such as urine testing, the client inferred that it wasn't important. Second, monitoring allows the provider to catch difficulties that the client may be having with the regimen, and to evaluate their relation to any changes in health status. Problem solving can then be jointly undertaken to reduce these difficulties by adjusting either the regimen or the client's behavior (or both). Third, monitoring provides the opportunity to reinforce and encourage the client to continue his or her efforts.

The importance of monitoring is supported by Svarstad's (1976) study of client visits with eight physicians. Svarstad reports than when clients were regularly asked if they had taken each drug, how many tablets they were taking daily, and how much medication was left in the container, 52% conformed to their medication regimens. In contrast, only 26% conformed who were asked in general terms whether they were taking their medications. Monitoring is more effective when done in a focused manner. If the client has kept records of regimen-following behavior, as suggested in the preceding section, these records can be reviewed by the provider.

The provider's role is to support the client in as nonjudgemental a way as possible. At those inevitable times when the client forgets to follow the regimen or other mistakes occur, the provider can help put them in perspective for the client. For example, a provider might have the client examine the progress he or she has made over time in handling specific situations or regimens. The provider also can help the client problem-solve what could be done differently the next time around. The emphasis, according to both Steckel (1981) and Ormiston (1980), should be on the client's success.

Problem Solving

Problem solving is an essential part of being able to respond to client's needs. More affectionately known as "the six steps to heaven,"[1] problem solving is a structured process by which an existing or potential problem is identified and examined in detail, so that a strategy for resolving the problem can be selected. The process is integral to designing and revising the regimen and to responding to the quality of life problems which the client raises. While at first the provider may simply model the problem-solving process, one approach to encouraging self-management is to involve the client more actively in the process over several visits.

There are several steps in this process; each of the steps is briefly discussed here and demonstrated with an example. The steps may be defined as follows: 1) problem formulation; 2) identification of alternate strategies; 3) evaluation of the alternatives; 4) development of an action plan; 5) anticipating problems; and 6) evaluation.

---

[1] This phrase belongs to colleague Jerry Rose, Center for Health Systems Research and Analysis, University of Wisconsin-Madison.

Problem formulation (Step 1). The goal of the first step of problem
solving, problem formulation, is to identify what the client perceives to be
the real problem. At times, the problem as identified by the client is closer
to a desired solution than an actual problem statement. It is usually
necessary for the provider to explore the client's problem definition
carefully. This needs to be done in a way that validates the client's sense
that his or her perceptions are important and that the provider does indeed
hear them. One approach is to write down the concern in the client's own
words, and then indicate that it is an important concern to work on together.
Even if the provider eventually must help the client reframe his or her
definition of the problem, this process of validation is a critical step.

Let's look at an example. A 19-year-old client, diagnosed six months
earlier as having insulin-dependent diabetes, is talking with her nurse. The
client feels she must change jobs because her present unpredictable schedule
at work makes it difficult to follow her regimen. Although the nurse feels
the problem was stated in the form of a solution (change jobs), she takes the
client's statement as an important first step in defining the problem. The
nurse writes down the problem as the client states it; then she asks the
client to talk about the pro's and con's of quitting the job. The nurse jots
the comments down in two different columns which the client can see. As they
talk, it becomes clearer to the nurse that the client is embarrassed about
having diabetes. She hopes that by changing jobs people at work will never
learn that she has diabetes. However, on the con side, the client also points
out that if she quits her job she will lose touch with close friends at her
current job.

After the list is completed the nurse asks the client which are the most
important issues in the two columns. The nurse then tries to communicate to
the client what she has heard by saying something like the following:

> "these are the things that I am hearing you say are
> probably the most important, because...[here the nurse
> restates the client's perception of the problem.] I'm also
> concerned from talking with you about...too [and here the
> nurse restates an aspect of the problem different from the
> client's statement]. How does this strike you?"

From this give-and-take process the client identifies her own embarrassment
about diabetes as one of the major problems.

Identifying alternatives (Step 2). The second step in the problem-solving
process is identifying a range of alternatives to solve the stated problem.
In our example, the 19-year-old generated several alternatives that were
recorded in writing by the nurse: quitting her job; talking just with her
immediate supervisor about the schedule constraints that her regimen imposed;
stopping her pre-lunch urine testing and reducing her insulin injections from
two to one in the morning; asking for a leave of absence while she attempted
both to get better control of her diabetes and also to become more comfortable
talking with friends about diabetes; joining a small group for
insulin-dependent diabetics in order to become more comfortable; taking a
vacation; and confiding in a few of her closest friends at work so that she

might trade a few of the least time-predictable tasks with them. As in the problem formulation step, the nurse writes down each strategy in the client's words so that the client can see the list, and then suggests a few other alternatives.

Evaluation of alternatives (Step 3). In the third step, evaluation of alternatives, the problem-solver considers the pro's and con's of each alternative developed and selects the most appealing alternative. In our example, two of the alternatives seem most useful to the client--reducing the urine-testing regimen and joining a small group. She also thinks she might discuss the problem with her supervisor but isn't sure she is up to that just yet, since she fears that her supervisor might over react. The nurse expresses her concern about reducing the urine testing schedule at this point, but feels that some compromise is certainly possible. The client decides to test her urine less frequently and also to join a small group for individuals with diabetes.

Developing an action plan (Step 4). The fourth step of the process is development of an action plan. In our example, the nurse and client design a schedule which varies from day to day for meals, snacks, and urine testing. On days the client feels would be more predictable she will do the full set of urine tests scheduled; on three of the workdays she will do reduced testing. The plan requires that she keep accurate records; these will be discussed at the following visit in three weeks. In addition, plans are made for the client to join a small group sponsored by the State Diabetes Association. The client decides she will not talk to her supervisor yet.

Anticipating problems (Step 5). In the fifth step of the process, anticipating problems, the nurse asks the client what she thinks might interfere with carrying out the plans she had just made. The client feels that the only problem might be with urine testing before noon on the two workdays; however, she hopes she can time her break enough before lunch to allow her to do the urine testing. To reinforce the young woman's sense of control, the nurse encourages her to try, but emphasizes that they can rethink the plan at the next visit if she has problems. The nurse asks the client to record her urine test results over the next three weeks so that they can discuss them during the next visit; she also indicates that if the client is concerned about her test values in the interim, she should call. She gives the client a specific time during the day that is best for receiving calls.

Evaluation (Step 6). In the sixth step, evaluation, the client and nurse use the next visit to evaluate the plan. They discuss whether any changes are needed in the plan, using the client's record of daily urine test results and of problems which interfered with the testing. Although the client wasn't able to record the values as consistently as she had hoped, the test results indicate fairly good control and she decides to continue with the plan for at least a few more weeks.

Summary. In this particular example, the client is very active in each step of the problem-solving process. In practice, there are times when it is hard for the client to do more than state a general problem and hard for the provider to do such detailed and highly-structured problem solving. At such times the provider may have to take responsibility for suggesting alternatives and helping the client weigh pro's and con's of the various alternatives. Nonetheless, even in this situation progress can be made by modeling a process that clients will go through more actively in the future.

COMMUNICATION ISSUES

The way information is collected and communicated influences how open clients will be and how satisfied they are with the care and advice they receive. Openness and satisfaction, in turn, affect how successfully regimens can be devised and revised. A growing number of researchers report that the provider's manner significantly affects not only satisfaction but also adherence. For example, clients were found to be less satisfied and also less adherent when providers did not give them feedback in response to information gathered (Davis, 1968; Korsch and Negrete, 1972). Apparently the interactive quality of history-taking is important to clients.

Provider affect--words, tone of voice, and body language--also seems to influence client outcomes significantly. In work by Davis (1968) verbal communication between physicians and clients was analyzed for its affective qualities. Clients were less adherent when physicians behaved in a way that might be interpreted as antagonistic, unless tension was released through joking or laughter. Without this tension release, patient cooperation with medical regimens decreased. Korsch and her colleagues (1972) also found that expression of negative affect (hostility, tension, punitiveness) by the physician reduced the client's adherence significantly. The manner in which information is collected and responded to by the provider can impact upon the client's satisfaction as well as subsequent efforts to adhere to the regimen.

The need for providers to be aware how their affective messages impact on clients was reinforced in work by Svarstad (1976) who found that 78% of the clients who received both high instruction and high friendliness from their providers conformed to the medication regimens prescribed for them. In contrast, only 42% of clients receiving high instruction, but low friendliness, conformed to the prescribed regimens. Providers who strive to be both warm and informative will be more effective in promoting client self-management of medications. Svarstad also notes that two of the eight physicians tended to give their instructions in a demanding or authoritative manner and frequently did not respond to client complaints about their medications. The clients of these physicians were more likely to hide their nonadherence when the physician questioned them than were clients of other physicians.

Insight into the process by which clients read physician cues is provided by Hall (1981), who compared the voice tone with the affective content of the words uttered by clients and two female physicians during client visits. Panels of 144 judges rated the words and voice tone of physicians and clients on a number of scales including anger, anxiety, and sympathy. Raters found it hard to distinguish between tonal expressions of anxiety and anger by both the client or the physician, so ratings of the two expressions tended to be highly correlated with each other. This suggests that in client visits, as in other communication situations, anxiety or anger may be easily misinterpreted.

The second finding of interest is that while client contentment with the visit was higher when providers' words expressed less anxiety and more sympathy (as judged by panels), client contentment was also higher when the provider's affective tone of voice expressed more anger or anxiety. Hall felt that clients may have interpreted any expression of feeling by the two female physicians as a reflection of a serious concern for the client.

CONCLUSION

This chapter has examined the partnership between client and provider during the client visit. In the need to balance issues of quality of life against management of the condition, active involvement of clients in the design and adaptation of their regimens allows the provider to foster both parts of this balance. To attain active client involvement, providers will need to be sensitive to the manner in which they collect and give information to clients, for their tone is as important as the content of their words. For some clients, the best of interpersonal processes may not be enough to promote self-management. As discussed in Chapter 1, clients with a history of nonadherence, with more complex regimens, or with substantial stressors may need other strategies to augment the provider's efforts to involve the client during the visit. For these clients, as well as for those who seek a higher level of self-management, the following chapters discuss a variety of strategies that can be used to promote further self-management and adherence. These include contracting, self-monitoring, educational and support groups, family involvement, and telephone and mail contact.

REFERENCES

Becker, M. H., and Maiman, L. Strategies for enhancing patient compliance. J. of Community Health 6:113-133, Winter 1980.

Boyd, J. R., and others. Drug Defaulting II. Analysis on noncompliance patterns. Amer. J. of Hosp. Pharm. 31:485-491, 1974.

Davis, M. S. Variations in patients' compliance with doctors' advice: an empirical analysis of patterns of communication. Amer. J. of Public Health 58:274-288, Feb 1968.

Dunbar, J., and others. Behavioral strategies for improving compliance. In: Hayes, R. B., and others, editors. Compliance in Health Care. Baltimore: Johns Hopkins University Press, 1979, pp. 174-192.

Fink, D. Tailoring the consensual regimen. In: Sackett, D. L., and Haynes, R. B., editors. Compliance with Therapeutic Regimens. Baltimore: Johns Hopkins University Press, 1976, pp. 110-118.

Genther, R., and Anderson, R. Psychological Assessment Handbook. Augusta, Maine: Diabetes Control Project, Medical Care Development, Inc., 1981.

Green, L., and others. Development of randomized patient education experiments with urban poor hypertensives. Patient Counselling and Health Educ. 1:106-111, Winter/Spring 1979.

Hall, J., and others. Communication of affect between patient and physician. J. of Health and Soc. Behavior 22:8-30, Mar 1981.

_____ A critical review of the determinants of patient compliance with antihypertensive treatment. In: Sackett, D. L., and Haynes, R. B., editors. Compliance with Therapeutic Regimens. Baltimore: Johns Hopkins University Press, 1976, pp. 26-39.

Haynes, R. B. Strategies to improve compliance with referrals, appointments and prescribed medical regimens. In: Haynes, R. B., and others, editors. Compliance in·Health Care. Baltimore: Johns Hopkins University Press, 1979, pp. 121-143.

--- A review of tested interventions for improving compliance with antihypertensive treatment. In: Haynes, R. B., and others, editors. Patient Compliance To Prescribed Antihypertensive Medication Regimens: A Report to the National Heart, Lung, and Blook Institute. Washington: U.S. Department of Health and Human Services, Public Health Service, National Institutes of Health, October 1980, pp. 83-112. NIH Publication No. 81-2102.

Hogue, C. Nursing and compliance. In: Haynes, R. B., and others, editors. Compliance in Health Care. Baltimore: Johns Hopkins University Press, 1979, pp. 242-259.

Hulka, B. Patient-clinician interactions and compliance In: Haynes, R. B., and others, editors. Compliance in Health Care. Baltimore: Johns Hopkins University Press, 1979, pp. 63-77.

Korsch, B., and Negrete, V. Doctor-patient communication. Scientific Amer. 227:66-74, 1972.

Leventhal, H., and others. The common sense representation of illness danger. In: Rachman, S., ed. Medical Psychology. II, Pergamon Press, 1980.

Meyer, D. L. The Effects of Patients' Representations of High Blood Pressure on Behavior in Treatment. Ph.D. dissertation, University of Wisconsin-Madison, 1980.

Mullen, P. The (already) activated patient: an alternative to medicocentrism. In: Wendy Squyres, editor. Patient Education: An Inquiry Into the State of the Art. New York: Springer Publishing Co., 1980, pp. 281-298.

Ormiston, L. Self-management strategies. In: Wendy Squyres, editor. Patient Education: An Inquiry Into the State of the Art. New York: Springer Publishing Co., 1980, pp. 217-246.

Sackett, D. The magnitude of compliance and noncompliance. In: Sackett, D. L., and Haynes, R. B., editors. Compliance with Therapeutic Regimens. Baltimore: The Johns Hopkins University Press, 1976, pp. 9-25.

Steckel, S. B. Increasing adherence of outpatients to therapeutic regimens. Project Final Report. Ann Arbor: Veterans Administration, Health Services Research and Development Project #343, 1981.

Steckel, S. B., and Swain, M. A. Contracting with patients to improve compliance. Hospitals, 51:81-84, 1977.

Stone, G. Patient compliance and the role of the expert. J. of Soc. Issues 35:34-59, 1979.

Svarstad, B. Physician-patient communication and patient conformity with medical advice. In: David Mechanic, editor. The Growth of Bureaucratic Medicine. New York: John Wiley and Sons, 1976, pp. 220-238.

Zifferblatt, S., and Curry, P. Patient self-management of hypertension medication. In: Barofsky, I. editor. Medication Compliance: A Behavioral Approach: Thorofare, New Jersey: Charles B. Slack, Inc., 1977, pp. 77-94.

CHAPTER 4
ACTIVE CLIENT INVOLVEMENT

CONTRACTING

There has been growing interest in contracting as a strategy for involving clients in their own care. In contracting, clients, with provider help, identify specific behaviors they will perform between now and the next health-care visit. The behaviors typically compose a series of small steps leading toward the client's health goal. This process appears to help shape client behaviors and to enhance commitment to following a regimen, even during periods of minimal reinforcement from other sources.

In their key study of clients with hypertension, Steckel and Swain (1977) found that contracting can influence and assist clients in controlling their blood pressure. One hundred fifteen clients were followed for four visits; none of the clients who developed contracts dropped out of the program during this time, as contrasted with an 8% drop-out rate for clients receiving only routine care, and a startling 26% drop-out rate for clients who received educational pamphlets on hypertension in addition to their routine care. Contracting also had a positive effect on blood pressure. In the contracting group, blood pressure stabilized at a standard for control by the second visit, whereas blood pressure of clients who received the pamphlet and routine care or who received routine care alone continued to fluctuate considerably during the four visits. Steckel and Swain hypothesize that it was not sufficient for clients to have information about hypertension without also acquiring the skills to break the regimen into concrete behaviors that they could perform.

In a later study involving 400 clients with hypertension, diabetes, or rheumatoid arthritis, contracts were renegotiated at each visit with clinic nurses (Steckel, 1981). In return for rewards they selected themselves, clients agreed to such behaviors as taking their pills, smoking less, or keeping appointments. Over a three-year period, only 3% of the contracts were not followed. Preliminary analysis of the data for clients with hypertension showed that the diastolic blood pressure of clients who had contracts dropped twice as quickly as for those without contracts. There was also significantly more weight loss for the contracting clients. The two studies (Steckel and Swain, 1977; Steckel, 1981) together suggest that contracting can be a useful tool for helping clients adhere to behaviors that they feel they can follow.

A third study of contracting, conducted by Herje (1981), provides an interesting contrast to the Steckel and Swain work. In all of their previous work, Steckel and Swain stipulated a reward for the client, should he or she perform the designated behavior. In Herje's study of clients with chronic lower back pain, no reward was identified in clients' contracts.* This

_____
*The subject of rewards did come up informally: the provider might say something like, "If you succeed in this, what especially nice thing would you do for yourself?" The provider offered suggestions of self-rewards such as a walk in the arboretum or taking time for oneself in a special way.

study found that contracting clients made more short-term protective posture changes and did more low-back exercises than did noncontracting clients who received an educational intervention. Thus, it may well be that stipulating a specific reward is less important than jointly identifying concrete do-able behaviors and monitoring the client's progress across visits.

Key Components of Contracting

There is general agreement in the literature that to be effective contracts with clients should:

- Focus on the <u>behaviors</u> that lead to the goal, rather than focusing on the end goal <u>itself</u>.

- Identify small steps which the client believes he or she can realistically do between now and the next visit.

- Describe a set of step that are unique to or tailored to that particular client.

- Lead ultimately toward an end goal that matters to the client, over a series of contracts.

- Identify a means by which client behaviors can be recorded.

- Identify a reward that the client values, if rewards are involved.

Key to successful client contracts is the identification of small, realistic steps which the client can take to reach a given goal. At times the content of the contract may seem to be at so low a level as to afford little progress, but the steps do in time lead to the end goal. The important thing is to keep the client in care and to increase the opportunity for success in managing the condition. Over a series of visits the client and provider can then negotiate intermediate behaviors. Successful performance of these behaviors moves the client closer to his or her final health goal, and provides the chance to acknowledge and reinforce the client's progress.

Table 4 shows a variety of behaviors that clients might contract to do. Each behavior is a small step which leads to the longer-term health goals.

TABLE 4   STEPS FOR CONTRACTS

Condition	Examples of behaviors
1. Arthritis	-- Lie down once a day for a 5-minute rest.
2. COPD	-- Push a shopping basket the length of a shopping mall twice a week.
3. Diabetes	-- Test with clinitest and record values two times a day for two weeks.
4. Hypertension	-- Keep an appointment to see the provider again in two weeks.

At times a client may make little progress in meeting the contract. It is important at such times not only to renegotiate a more realistic contract, but also to reinforce the client for having kept his or her appointment despite the lack of progress. Some providers keep in reserve a surprise reward for clients who have not met contract goals but had the courage to return, anyway. This would not appear in the written contract.

One useful format for contracts stipulates the behavior to be performed by the client, the reward for following the contract, and the means of recording the behavior during the contract period (Steckel, 1980). A bonus reward clause to acknowledge large gains in progress may also be included (see Figure 2).

CONTRACT

I, _____, will _____ in return

for _____.

                     SIGNED _____ (Client)

                     SIGNED _____ (Provider)

                     DATED _____

Means of recording to be used: _____

Bonus Clause: _____

FIGURE 2. ESSENTIAL CONTRACT ELEMENTS

If rewards are used, clients need to select rewards which they think will help them adhere to the contract. While some people select material rewards such as money or lottery tickets, many choose rewards related to increased provider contact (e.g., a phone call, or more time at the next visit). Given the uniqueness of people in their needs and preferences, this aspect of the contract is best selected by the client, although staff may want to suggest a range of options to the client.

It is important to have some means of recording the contracted behaviors when they are performed, for example a blood pressure log, a food diary, an exercise diary (including time, date, kind, and duration), or a rest log (recording date and time). At the next visit the client and provider, each of whom has a copy of the contract, can examine the record in relation to the contract. Any difficulties in adhering to the contract can be discussed as part of the negotiation of the next contract. The client may wish to alter the contract with staff help, by either reducing or expanding the behaviors. From their work, Steckel and Swain recommend that maintenance contracts be continued after clients have reached their end goals. The contract still can serve its function of encouraging both client and provider to acknowledge and reinforce what the client is doing well.

Heightening the Effectiveness of Contracting

A limited number of studies have varied the conditions under which contracting is used, to identify ways of enhancing its effectiveness. Most of the studies suggest that providing additional reinforcement or support for following a contract is helpful. Etzwiler (1980), in a brief summary of research with diabetics, reports that adherence with urine testing over a two-week period was increased from 52% to 64% when staff called clients once during the two week period. It was increased to 80% when staff called clients twice. An increase of almost 30 percentage points was achieved through the relatively inexpensive means of two brief phone calls to remind clients of their urine testing contracts.

The weight-loss research provides more suggestions for practitioners. In a study of 106 overweight volunteers, Ureda (1980) found that having a friend or family member read and sign the client contract resulted in more reported client intention to adhere to regimens and in more weight loss than did having the client alone sign the contract. Saccone and Israel (1978) clarify further that having a significant other witness the contract reinforces the client's adherence attempts when the contract is for specific behaviors (e.g., not eating between meals), but not when it is directed to goals only, such as a specified number of pounds lost. The additional social attention to the contract appears to make a significant difference.

To summarize, three additional factors to consider when planning to use contracting are the ability of staff to design structured, behavior-specific contracts such as those modeled by Steckel (1981), the possibility of occasional telephone follow-up to check the client progress, and the feasibility of having a client's contract witnessed by a significant other chosen by the client.

Client and Staff Perceptions

How do clients perceive contracting, as opposed to a more traditional patient-education intervention? Research by Schulman (1979, 1980) is relevant to this issue. Working with the same population as in Steckel and Swain's earlier (1977) study of clients with hypertension, more clients who developed contracts reported they were involved as participants in their care than did clients without contracts. They also reported that staff gave them more facts and educational resources. The authors indicate that contracting clients more than noncontracting clients commented on the guidance they were given in putting the facts to use and in carrying out medical recommendations. It is interesting that all the clients, including those in a contracting group, were only mildly interested in having input into decisions pertaining to their treatment.

Clients' belief that staff encouraged them to be active participants was as important for predicting the study's outcomes as whether clients were in the group that actually developed contracts. Specifically, clients' bloodpressure control, self-reported adherence, and beliefs about the treatment's value were related highly to their belief that they had been active participants, regardless of whether they signed a contract. A valuable point which the authors make about this finding is that some clients seek and receive more information and involvement regardless of whether a contract is involved. For some people, active involvement comes easily. Contracting is one technique that helps to structure the visit so that all clients have this opportunity. As the Schulman research suggests, contracting itself may not be as important as the client's perception that he or she was treated as an active partner or participant in the care process.

There is evidence that providers also find the contracting satisfying. Hefferin (1979) examined staff perceptions of the contracting process. According to Hefferin, nurses reported significantly more satisfaction in working with clients who formed contracts. They were more satisfied with their assessment, care planning, sharing client-care information, and receiving feedback on the client's progress from the client.

Steckel reports that some providers are uncomfortable using the technique of contracting because they view it as manipulative. For this reason it is important for providers to be clear about their own feelings before doing contracting. As Steckel points out, tangible rewards such as money or books need not be used. In fact, many clients prefer receiving extra time with staff as a reward. The Herje research further suggests that rewards may be much less important than other elements of the contracting process, e.g., focusing on behaviors which the client can and wants to follow.

System Costs of Contracting

A visit that includes the process of negotiating contracts with patients takes about 12 minutes (Steckel and Swain, 1977). Staff orientation would involve an initial investment of time. Hefferin (1979) reports having used four one-hour sessions to orient 50 nurses new to the contracting process. The types of rewards offered to patients will also influence the costs of using contracting with clients. For example, a common intangible but not cost-free reward is five minutes extra with a staff member at the next visit; another is a weekly telephone call at an appointed time. With more tangible rewards, additional costs will vary with the nature of the reward.

MEDICAL RECORDS

As Schulman (1979) points out, often people receiving health care do not view themselves as rightful and necessary parties to treatment plans and activities. But, for the control of chronic conditions in particular, their active participation is critical. For this reason a range of strategies to support this participation should be considered. Contracting is one such strategy; another is client co-authoring of the medical record. Although only pilot research has been done on medical record co-authoring, it provides interesting qualitative information about the effects of involving clients actively during the visit.

A pilot study by Fishbach and Sionelo-Bayog (1980) investigated the usefulness of having clients with chronic conditions collaborate with their health care providers in co-authoring their medical records at each visit. Their research suggests that having the client and physician complete the record jointly can result in more complete and mutually understandable information. The sample included 24 people with mild to severe hypertension, diabetes mellitus, and/or congestive heart failure.

Key Components of Medical Record Use

In the Fishbach and Sionelo-Bayog study (1980), a typical visit began with the client formulating a problem list, with the provider at times suggesting modifications before placing it in the medical record. The client and provider together then wrote a continuation note that included the client's symptoms, clinical findings, and assessment. They then designed a plan tailored specifically to the needs of the client; this could function informally as a contract, describing the obligations and responsibilities of each. Clients kept copies of the co-authored medical record and plan, along with home monitoring records and patient education materials, in a notebook brought to each clinic visit.

No effort was made to conduct a statistical analysis on this pilot project, but the impressions recorded by researchers and staff have practical implications for clinicians. Although initially clients were very diffident, gradually they became more active and constructive partners, focusing on more relevant symptoms and recording key information at home. The joint writing process helped eliminate serious client misconceptions about the condition and its management and extended the provider's opportunity to assess the client's knowledge and attitudes. There was also marked improvement in appointment keeping.

Another study that used medical record information to involve clients, this time in a university health setting, supports the usefulness of a medical records strategy (Giglio and others, 1978). Although the small sample size (35) limits the conclusions which can be drawn, clients reported significantly more involvement in their own health and adherence to recommended behaviors.

Client and Provider Perceptions

Clients in the Fishbach study were described as very attached to their record books; they would bring them to visits with providers not involved in the study. All of the clients remained with the study. After the study ended, the staff and clients continued their new roles rather than returning to their traditional provider-"patient" relationship. The lack of self-confidence that marked the client role early in the study was replaced with active client participation by the end. Similar patterns were reported by the Giglio (1978) study. There, the clients initially were somewhat unsure or apprehensive about changing their roles to assume a more equal partnership with the provider; however, by the end of the project this self-consciousness about roles decreased and clients accepted primary responsibility for their own health and its maintenance.

Both studies indicated that at first providers (primarily physicians) were very anxious about using the medical record to promote active client participation in the visit and to design their care plan. Fishbach and Sionelo-Bayog (1980) point out that joint authorship for the provider meant "adopting a new writing style, a delicate balance in trying to be concise without resorting to ambiguity or euphemisms while simultaneously recording anxiety-provoking material." The authors report that despite their initial skepticism providers were able to benefit from an improved communication process. They were relieved to find that their worst fears were not confirmed, in that "too much" information did not make clients either too anxious or too directive. The providers' fear that their practice would be judged deficient from record audits also decreased.

Costs of Medical Record Involvement

Initially, as both the provider and client became accustomed to their new roles, client-provider interactions took as much as 50% longer. Fishbach and Sionelo-Bayog (1980) estimate that 15-20% of physician time with clients was spent orienting them to the new process. Thus, clearly there is an early outlay of staff time in orienting clients, developing a shared language, and developing a writing style that is clear and direct for clients. Fishbach believes that the initial investment of staff time is more than compensated by the increased efficiency of the client's future visits.

REFERENCES

Etzwiler, D. D. Teaching allied health professionals about self-management. Diabetes Care 3:121-123, Jan 1980.
Fishbach, R., Sionelo-Bayog, A. The patient and practitioner as co-authors of the medical record. Patient Counselling and Health Educ. 2:1-5, First Quarter, 1980.

Giglio, R., and others. Encouraging behavior changes by use of client-held health records. Med. Care 16:757-764, Sept 1978.

Hefferin, E. A. Health goal setting: patient-nurse collaboration at Veterans Administration facilities. Military Med. 144:814-822, Dec 1979.

Herje, P. A. Behavioral contracting with persons with low back pain: An experimental study. Masters Thesis, University of Wisconsin-Madison, 1981.

Saccone, A. J. and Israel, A. Effects of experimenter versus significant other controlled reinforcement and choice of target behavior on weight loss. Behavior Therapy 9:271-278, Mar 1978.

Schulman, B. A. Active patient orientation and outcomes in hypertension treatment. Med. Care 17:267-279, Mar 1979.

Schulman, B. A., and Swain, M. A. Active patient orientation. Patient Counselling and Health Educ. 2:32-37, First Quarter, 1980.

Steckel, S. B. Contracting with patient-selected reinforcers. Amer. J. of Nurs. 80:1596-1599, Sept. 1980.

Steckel, S. B. Increasing adherence of outpatients to therapeutic regimens. Project Final Report. Ann Arbor: Veterans Administration, Health Services Research and Development Project #343, 1981.

Steckel, S. B., and Swain, M. A. Contracting with patients to improve compliance. Hospitals 51:81-84, Dec 1977.

Swain, M. A., and Steckel, S. B. Influencing adherence among hypertensives. Res. in Nurs. and Health 4:213-222, Mar 1981.

Ureda, J. R. The effect of contract witnessing on motivation and weight loss in a weight control program. Health Educ. Quarterly 7:163-185, Fall 1980.

CHAPTER 5
SELF-MONITORING HYPERTENSION AND DIABETES

HOME BLOOD PRESSURE MONITORING

Research on home blood pressure measurement suggests that, except for clients at clear risk for nonadherence, home blood pressure measurement has only a modest impact on lowering clients' blood pressure. However, for clients with a history of nonadherence or who anticipate having trouble remembering their medications, home blood pressure monitoring does appear to promote adherence, particularly when combined with other interventions (Baranowski and others, 1978; Carnahan and others, 1975; Haynes and others, 1976; Johnson and others, 1978; Nessman and others, 1980; Ogbuokiri, 1980).

The clearest findings in this regard are provided in a study of 39 nonadherent Canadian steelworkers who, after six months of treatment, had not achieved a diastolic blood pressure of 95 mm Hg (Haynes and others, 1976). To test whether their adherence and blood pressure could be improved, this group was taught to measure their own blood pressure and to tailor their regimens to the rituals and cues of their daily lives. In addition, they returned every two weeks for blood pressure checks and received $4 credit toward ownership of the home blood pressure cuff if the check was either 90 mm Hg or 4 mm Hg below that observed at the sixth month. By the end of this second six months the nonadhering group of clients had reduced diastolic blood pressure an additional 5.4 mm Hg, approaching the average fall observed among highly adhering clients at the first six months.

In a second study by this same research group, blood pressure monitoring had a positive effect on blood pressure only for clients who reported at the outset of treatment that they thought they would have difficulty remembering their medications (Johnson and others, 1978). Thus, home blood pressure monitoring does seem to be a tool that can help clients who expect, or have a history of, nonadherence.

It is important to note that clinicians may wish to use home blood pressure monitoring to promote outcomes besides adherence. Recent research suggests that clients often believe they know whether their blood pressure is elevated or normal (Meyer, 1980; Leventhal and others, 1980). Unfortunately, clients tend to have their blood pressure checked only when they believe it is high, and therefore they rarely validate their own subjective evaluation that it is low. For these clients, regular home blood pressure measurement can foster a more realistic perception of their own blood pressure patterns.

Studies in this area raise at least as many questions as they answer. One such question, relevant to discussions of adherence strategies in general, is whether it is realistic to expect a single intervention, such as blood pressure monitoring, to improve adherence and blood pressure when it is introduced alone. Haynes and others (1980) maintain that it is not realistic and suggests that we should be identifying the unique combination of interventions that makes the most sense for the particular client and for the resources of the health setting. The most positive findings regarding home blood pressure measurement occurred when it was introduced in combination with other strategies, such as home visits (Earp and Ory, 1979), frequent clinic visits with monetary reinforcement and regimens tailored to the client's lifestyle (Haynes and others, 1976), or client participation in small groups for support (Nessman and others, 1980; Ziesat, 1978).

At this point it is difficult to say what causes the positive impact of adherence strategies such as home blood pressure monitoring. While it may be something inherent in the strategy, the positive impact may simply be an effect of the increased attention that clients receive. Home blood pressure monitoring provides a convenient means for giving the client this attention in a focused way at each visit.

Key Components

Even though many questions remain to be answered with respect to home blood pressure monitoring, the published research and clinical experience do suggest a number of recommendations that are organized under the headings of assessment and method.

Assessment. In deciding whether to teach a client home blood pressure measurement, assess the following. Does the client:

- Expect to have trouble remembering his or her medications?

- Have a history of nonadherence?

- Believe he or she knows when blood pressure is elevated? (If yes, blood pressure measurements can help the client establish the accuracy of his or her perception that it is high or low.)

- Seem highly nervous or preoccupied with small changes in blood pressure (2 mm Hg)? (If yes, blood pressure measurement may aggravate the preoccupation.)

- Want to learn self-blood pressure measurement skills?

Method. In teaching blood pressure measurement:

- First demonstrate self-measurement on yourself, so that the client sees how it is done, and sees that even staff require a bit of dexterity. Let the client listen to your sounds and take your blood pressure.

---

[1] See Consumer Reports, March 1979, for a good evaluation of blood pressure kits in terms of convenience, accuracy, and cost. Clients as well as staff may be interested in reading this.

. Then have the client take his or her own blood pressure and
  listen to the sounds. (Warn the client not to pump with the
  hand that has the cuff on it.)

. Warn clients not to take their first few home readings too
  seriously and to return within 1-2 weeks so that their
  readings can be checked.

. Consider lending a stethoscope and cuff to the client initially
  while he or she decides about buying their own equipment.[1]

. If the client does choose to buy the equipment, staff should
  check the accuracy of the equipment so that if necessary a
  replacement can be made before the warranty runs out.

. Encourage clients to take and record their readings at
  regular times during the week.

. Set aside time at the beginning of each visit to review the
  client's recorded blood pressure readings. This provides an
  opportunity to offer support, note any values that seem
  elevated, and explore with the client why any elevated
  readings might have occurred.

The clinicians we interviewed indicated that clients usually can say
whether they want to measure their own blood pressure. Because at some point
clients have to decide for or against purchase, a self-selection process
occurs and only the more interested clients continue monitoring their blood
pressure.

Client and Staff Perceptions

Clients respond favorably to home blood pressure monitoring. Out of 70
people monitoring their own blood pressure in one study, 90% thought it was
useful and 88% said they did not feel more anxious about their blood pressure
as a result of using a cuff (Johnson, 1978). In a separate study (Glanz and
others, 1981a; 1981b), 41% of the clients taking their blood pressure reported
it increased how much they thought about their high blood pressure, and 86%
percent reported that it was interesting to take their own blood pressure.
Only 30% reported it took some trouble to do home monitoring, as compared with
46% who reported that it took some trouble to keep a diary of medications
consumed.

Staff who were interviewed about client self-blood pressure monitoring
indicated that some clients were very interested in measuring their blood
pressure. For those clients, self-monitoring was an important aspect of the
self-management program. Providers found it particularly useful when clients
kept records of their values, which were reviewed at each visit. The records
offered a concrete way to examine how the client had been doing, problem-solve
around specific problems, and reinforce the client's active role in managing
the condition.

System Costs

Clinicians estimate that it takes approximately 15 minutes to teach a client how to measure blood pressure. In succeeding visits it is useful to take a few minutes during the history-taking to gather the client's home blood pressure readings.

The clinic may wish to purchase a few stethoscopes and blood pressure cuffs to lend to clients (typically for a few weeks). The provider may be able to purchase these at cost, particularly if the health care setting already purchases a large quantity of supplies from this source.

BLOOD GLUCOSE MONITORING

Published research on the impact of blood glucose self-monitoring is limited largely to case studies and evaluation of programs involving small numbers of clients with diabetes. Therefore, only preliminary inferences can be drawn. Nevertheless, these case studies consistently suggest that, especially for young adults and high risk populations (clients who are pregnant or have retinal disease), home blood glucose monitoring can help clients to control their blood sugar levels and can aid the general task of self-management (Dupuis and others, 1980; Irsigler and Ball-Taubald, 1980; Peterson and others, 1979).

Key Components

An invaluable feature of home blood glucose monitoring is that it provides immediate and precise feedback to people about their own metabolic balance. The primary drawbacks to blood glucose self-monitoring are its cost and the frequency with which readings must, at least initially, be taken. Assessment can help determine whether it is appropriate for a particular client to do self-monitoring via blood glucose, given that urine testing is much less expensive and provides sufficient accuracy for most purposes.

Tattersall (1980) and his colleagues regard home blood glucose monitoring as most appropriate for "brittle diabetic" clients (i.e., any clients having problems with diabetic control, pregnant diabetic women, and clients who have just started to make a serious effort to achieve normoglycemia). In addition, some clients, already highly motivated, may wish to take advantage of any technique that can enhance their blood glucose control. Clinicians who we interviewed believe that the blood glucose monitoring technique should be made available to this group as well, if they want it. Otherwise, urine testing continues to be a cheaper and satisfactory alternative for clients who do not need to adjust their insulin doses frequently and who understand how their metabolism fluctuates with diet and exercise. Health care providers working with clients monitoring their blood glucose, note that clients have to be motivated and facile at reading and interpreting the blood values. Some clients are clearly more able to learn this skill than others.

If the decision is made by client and provider to proceed with home glucose monitoring the following steps are recommended:

. Staff (nurse, physician's assistant, physician) will need to spend a visit preparing the person to do testing and diary recording. Often the company selling major equipment for blood glucose monitoring will want to train clients who will be using their equipment.[2]

. In addition to the blood glucose record, the client should also keep a diary of food and exercise in relation to the times at which blood glucose is measured.

. For a minimum of two weeks the client should take 6-8 blood sugar measurements daily--before each meal, 1-2 hours following a meal, and before going to bed.

. Within at least two weeks, follow-up should be done to correct any errors and help the client interpret the results. Monthly visits should continue until staff and the client are confident of the client's ability to read and interpret the values.

. Set aside time at the beginning of each visit to review the client's recorded blood glucose values. This provides an opportunity to offer support, note any values outside the normal range, and explore with the client why these readings might have occurred and how to establish better control.

With this rapid feedback system, a person can learn fairly quickly how deviations from normal activity, diet, and insulin regimen affect blood glucose levels. At the same time that clients are learning their body's own parameters, they are receiving very clear reinforcement for adhering to regimens that provide control of their blood glucose levels.

To reduce the cost of the stix and meter for reading blood glucose values, it is possible to have some clients monitor blood glucose levels for a two week period once a year (though also at times when blood glucose is expected to fluctuate, such as on holidays or during illness); for the rest of the year, these clients would rely on urine testing. Meters cost from $300 to $400. Some clinics purchase the meters for periodic use by clients. When precision is required, as with pregnant women, metered systems are appropriate. However, in other circumstances, visual interpretation of blood glucose values is usually accurate enough, providing that the client can detect color differences and interpolate values correctly (Reeves and others, 1981). The stix cost about 45 - 60¢ apiece. With 6-8 tests daily, this can become expensive. Clients who wish to continue monitoring blood glucose levels after readings have stabilized may reduce their readings to three a day. (Skyler and others, 1981).

---

[2] See Consumer Reports, June 1982, for a description of new home techniques for blood glucose monitoring, steps in use, and cost. Clients as well as staff may be interested in reading this.

Client and Staff Perspectives

The published testimonials from clients who are monitoring their blood glucose levels are remarkably enthusiastic (Patient Panel, 1980). Staff likewise report that the client response is very positive (Dupuis, 1980; Irsigler and Ball-Taubald, 1980; Peterson, 1979). Clients report that the procedure can be incorporated into the daily routine fairly easily, and that it is less distasteful and disruptive than urine testing. One client's response shows the immediacy of the link between feedback and motivated adherence:

> "I felt that a whole new world of freedom and information was available to me. I ate according to my blood sugar. If I was high, I didn't eat. If I was low, I ate. The measurement seemed to fill that gap of information that I had been looking for. I was able to see the interaction of insulin and food and activity and the resulting effects on blood sugar levels, and I can now apply those principles more effectively."

Thus far the method has been tested mostly with populations that are highly motivated—clients with retinopathy problems, or pregnant clients. It will be important to evaluate its use with clients whose risk and motivation are less.

One of the early concerns about the use of home blood glucose monitoring had been that clients might become depressed or even obsessed with their blood levels, since the measurement would be done so many times a day. However, Dupuis and his co-workers (1980) found that not only did self-monitoring of blood glucose lead to better management of the blood glucose levels, but that the emotional status of clients improved over the course of their self monitoring. For instance, clients reported feeling much more in control than they had at first, when using urine testing.

The literature is very positive about introducing blood glucose monitoring to clients. Our interviews with providers confirm that, aside from reservations about the cost of the procedure, they seem optimistic that it can be useful for at least a subset of clients. This was particularly true for providers who tend to see clients at the point when complications have begun to develop.

System Costs

The initial teaching session with patients takes an estimated 30-40 minutes of staff time. This can be done by nurses or physician's assistants (Skyler and others, 1980). Often companies selling major blood glucose monitoring equipment will conduct training sessions for clients. Follow-up by providers is advised two weeks after the client has begun the process. If clients have major medical insurance coverage, they can sometimes get 80% of the blood glucose monitoring cost covered. Clients without such coverage, however, often cannot afford the meters (costing $250-$400). Clinics may thus choose to buy this equipment to lend or rent to clients, although such a procedure leaves the clinic somewhat vulnerable to additional repair and calibration costs.

Given the costs to the client and/or clinic if meters are purchased, it is interesting to note the hospital cost savings that Irsigler and Ball-Taubald (1980) identified in their study of 17 pregnant women. Comparing pregnant diabetic women from 1978 with those doing blood glucose monitoring, his study revealed hospitalization was reduced by 45 days for the latter group. Clients learned to react quickly in order to correct slight fluctuations of blood glucose levels; this resulted in reduced hospitalization days and costs over the period of gestation.

REFERENCES

Baranowski, R., and others. A rural mining community high blood pressure control project. A paper presented at a Poster Session of the National Conference on High Blood Pressure Control, Los Angeles, California, April 3, 1978.

Carnahan, J., and others. The effects of self-monitoring by patients on the control of hypertension, Amer. J. of the Med. Sci. 269(1):69-73, Jan-Feb 1975.

Blood Pressure Kits. Consumer's Reports 44:142-146, Mar 1979.

Dupuis, A., and others. Assessment of the psychological factors and responses in self-managed patients. Diabetes Care 3:117-119, Jan/Feb 1980.

Earp, J., and Ory, M. The effects of social support and health professional home visits on patient adherence to hypertension regimens. A paper presented at the National Conference on High Blood Pressure Control, Washington, D.C., April 6, 1979.

Glanz, K., and others. Linking research and practice in patient education for hypertension patient responses to four educational interventions. Med. Care 19:141-152, Feb 1981.

Glanz, K., and others. Initial knowledge and attitudes as predictors of intervention effects: the individual management plan. Patient Counselling and Health Educ. 3:30-42, First Quarter 1981.

Haynes, R. B., and others. Improvement of medication compliance in uncontrolled hypertension. The Lancet 1:1265-1268, Jun 1976.

Haynes, R. B., and others. A review of tested interventions for improving compliance with antihypertensive treatment. In: Patient Compliance to Prescribed Antihypertensive Medication Regimens: A Report to the National Heart, Lung, and Blood Institute. Washington: U.S. Department HHS, Public Health Service, National Institutes of Health, October 1980, 139-164 NIH Publication No. 81-2102.

Irsigler, K., and Ball-Taubald, C. Self-monitored blood glucose: the essential feedback signal in the diabetic patient's effort to achieve normoglycemia. Diabetes Care 3:163-170, Jan/Feb 1980.

Johnson, A., and others. Self-recording of blood pressure in the management of hypertension. Can. Med. Assoc. J. 119:1034-1039, Nov 1978.

Leventhal, H., and others. The common sense representation of illness danger. In: Rachman, S., editor. Contributions to Medical Psychology. Vol. II. New York: Pergamon, 1980, pp. 7-30.

Meyer, D. The Effects of Patients' Representations of High Blood Pressure on Behavior in Treatment. Ph.D. dissertation, University of Wisconsin-Madison, 1980.

Nessman, D., and others. Increasing compliance in patient operated hypertension groups. Arch. of Intern. Med. 140:1427-1430, Nov 1980.

New Tests to Monitor Diabetes at Home. Consumer's Reports 47:318-320, Jun 1982.

Obguorkiri, J. E. Self-monitoring of blood pressure in hypertensive subjects and its effects on patient compliance. Drug Intelligence and Clinical Pharmacy 14:424-427, Jun 1980.

Patient Panel. Diabetes Care 3:144-149, Jan./Feb 1980.

Peterson, C. M., and others. Feasibility of improved blood glucose control in patients with insulin-dependent diabetes mellitus. Diabetes Care 2:329-335, Jul/Aug 1979.

Reeves, M. S., and others. Comparison of methods for blood glucose monitoring. Diabetes Care 4:404-406, May/Jun 1981.

Skyler, J., and others. Algorithms for adjustment of insulin dosage by patients who monitor blood glucose. Diabetes Care 4:311-318, Mar/Apr 1981.

Tattersall, R., and others. A critical evaluation of methods of monitoring diabetic control. Diabetes Care 3:150-154, Jan/Feb 1980.

Ziesat, H. A. Behavioral modification in the treatment of hypertension. Int. J. of Psychiat. in Med. 8:247-265, 1978.

CHAPTER 6
SMALL GROUPS

The use of small groups has been viewed by many as an effective way to
provide clients with both educational and emotional support. Self-management
of a chronic condition requires not only mastery of specific skills to control
the condition, but also an emotional adjustment to follow regimens and
possibly make lifestyle changes. The literature on small groups suggests that
sharing insights and feelings with peers can help clients adjust to and manage
their conditions (Ashikaga and others, 1980; Dupuis, 1980; Green and others,
1977; Levine and others, 1979; Lorig and others, 1981; Nessman and others,
1980; Peterson and Jones, 1979; Syme, 1977; Ziesat, 1977).

This literature contains a wide variety of models for how small groups can
be structured. Unfortunately, as Levy (1980) points out in her review of the
hypertension small-group research, much of this literature describes group
content and structure in such general terms that it is difficult to infer
exactly what aspect of the group process led to its impact. To compensate for
this deficit, this chapter will examine a subset of studies in more detail.

The following section compares the structure and outcomes of small groups
in five studies to provide several examples of how small groups can be
organized. It is hoped that this will help readers design small groups
appropriate to their client population. The five small-group models to be
discussed have been chosen for their range of client populations and for their
differences in process and structure; all five include a control group of
nonparticipants to compare against small-group participants. Each of the
small groups will be contrasted on: 1) intensity of the intervention (duration
and number of meetings); 2) extent of family involvement; 3) relative mix of
education and social support; and 4) specific strategies used to promote
adherence. The comparison is summarized in Table 6.

An interesting group model for people with arthritis is offered by Lorig
and others (1981). The group intervention consists of fourteen hours of
arthritis self-management education given in four weekly sessions of two hours
each followed by three additional two hour sessions one month apart. Trained
lay co-leaders present principles of self-management in the first quarter of
the session; then participants break into pairs or small groups to apply the
principles to their own situation. For example, after principles of exercise
have been explained, participants break into pairs to develop their own
exercise plans. Since family are invited, pairs often include a significant
other, thus providing the basis for ongoing support. At the end of each
session participants return to the larger group to share their individual
plans. After 18 months, increased self-management, reduced pain, and fewer
clinic visits resulted for participants.

A second model is provided by Nessman and others (1980). Over eight
sessions, participants are given information about hypertension and its
management, discuss health beliefs, learn to measure their own blood pressure,
and then formulate their own regimen within standard diet and drug protocols.
After eight months, participants showed a significant drop in blood pressure,
and had better pill counts and clinic attendance than did nonparticipants.

TABLE 5. SMALL GROUP COMPARISONS

ASHIKAGA, 1980. COPD: 6 sessions, 2 hrs. each. Family invited.

Support/Education	Adherence Strategies	Outcomes
Divided sessions in half; information presented first, then discussion on problems of living with COPD followed.	Family included; skills practiced during sessions	After 4 months participants (compared to controls): 1. Increased self-help behaviors. 2. Increased readiness to seek health care when needed.

LEVINE, 1979. Hypertension: 3 sessions, 2 hrs. ea. No family involvement.

Support/Education	Adherence Strategies	Outcomes
Information not a goal. Group aimed at increasing participants' confidence in coping with their condition, controlling associated problems.	Participants made contract with group leader; took each other's blood pressure. Group problem-solved individual members' needs, then role-played solutions.	After 8 months: Percentage with controlled blood pressure increased significantly.

LORIG, 1981. Arthritis: 7 sessions, 2 hrs. ea. Family invited.

Support/Education	Adherence Strategies	Outcomes
At start of session, principles of self-management were presented. Social support was provided through small groups and pairing (which could include family).	Working in small groups or in pairs, participants (including family members) applied principles presented to their own situation. Practiced skills during sessions.	After 18 months participants (compared to controls): 1. Increased exercise, relaxation, contacts with others. 2. Made 1 to 1 1/2 fewer visits per year to doctor or clinic. 3. Reported less pain.

NESSMAN, 1980. Hypertension: 8 sessions, 90 min. ea. No family involvement.

Support/Education	Adherence Strategies	Outcomes
Information discussed on hypertension and drugs, including side effects. Members discussed seriousness of disease, perceived personal susceptibility, and their faith in and satisfaction with treatment.	Learned to measure own blood pressure; formulated own regimen (within standard diet and drug protocols).	After 8 months participants (compared to controls): 1. Had blood pressure drop significantly more. 2. Had significantly better pill counts and clinic attendance.

ZIESAT, 1977. Hypertension: 4 sessions (length not reported). Social ally was identified for support, but did not attend sessions.

Support/Education	Adherence Strategies	Outcomes
Early in sessions participants were educated about diet, medication, and self-monitoring.	Blood pressure was recorded and reinforced at each session. Each member identified cues for taking medications. Peers instructed each other about regimen. Each identified an ally outside of group to help with adherence.	After 3 weeks: Diastolic blood pressure fell from 104.2 to 89.8 mm Hg.

Although teaching was a basic part of the effort to empower group participants in several models (Ashikaga and others, 1980; Lorig and others, 1981; Nessman and others, 1980; Ziesat, 1977), it was less important in the small-group model studied by Levine and colleagues (1979). In this study, the primary goal of the small groups was to increase clients' confidence and sense of control about managing their condition, rather than to teach them about specific aspects of the hypertension regimen. To accomplish this, participants first identified their individual needs and then established a contract with the group leader. During each session, members addressed individual needs through group problem-solving. After the group had generated a strategy to address an individual's problem, behavioral rehearsal and role playing was done to increase skills and confidence for carrying out the strategy. In addition, participants measured each other's blood pressure and discussed the implications of the recorded values. After eight months, the findings indicated that the percentage of clients with controlled blood pressure increased significantly for those who attended all three sessions.

A strongly behavioral model is offered in a study by Ziesat (1977). At the beginning of each session, each participant's blood pressure was measured, recorded, and reinforced in front of the group. Each member identified daily cues for taking medications, and participants consulted with each other in pairs about regimens. In addition, each member identified a social ally outside of the group to reinforce his or her adherence efforts. The study found that participants' blood pressure dropped from a mean of 104.2 to 89.8 mm Hg in three weeks. Unfortunately, there was no long-term blood pressure measurement to evaluate the longer-term effects of the intervention, and the number of small group participants was small.

The small-group structure and process tends to vary by participants' chronic conditions. Groups designed for clients with hypertension tend to emphasize education and adherence more than emotional support, while groups for participants with arthritis and COPD tend to allow more time for participants to discuss problems in daily living, and to exchange insights and support. This is seen in the small-group model for clients with COPD studied by Ashikaga and colleagues (1980). The first hour was spent learning and practicing self-help techniques such as relaxation and diaphragmatic breathing. In the second hour, participants and family members discussed their concerns. Staff tried to stay in the background as much as possible and let participants direct the second hour's agenda. After four months, group participants had increased their self-help behaviors more than nonparticipants.

All five studies, despite variation in structure, report positive findings associated with group participation. However, there is a strong need for research to examine how specific variations of small group structure influence outcomes.

KEY COMPONENTS

In the absence of literature that supports definitive conclusions about key components of small groups, clinicians were contacted to identify key issues to consider when designing small groups. The following issues were identified in these conversations.

Criteria for Involvement

In deciding whether to encourage a client to participate in a group consider the following:

. What will the individual get out of the group relative to his or
  her needs for information, peer contact, support, and
  self-management help?

. What impact will the individual have on the group? . Will the individual bring the ability to share attention, support, and experience that will aid others?

. Will the individual help provide a good mix of group participants? It is important that the group have at least a few members who have already come to terms with their condition and have re-evaluated their priorities and assets. These members can often be extremely valuable in helping others confront a similar situation. Although this re-evaluation is rarely easy, it helps to see others who have discarded values and roles that are now dysfunctional.

. Is the person physically and emotionally able to participate in group activities? The physical condition of an individual may not permit certain types of exercise, diet, or other aspects of the small-group training. As protection for both the participant and the sponsor of the group, it is helpful for participants to get advice from their physician about attending if they have a regular source of care.

Designing The Group

Several issues must be addressed before and during the process of designing the group structure and schedule:

. Who should determine the group's priorities and objectives -- providers, clients, both? An informal needs assessment among clients can be extremely helpful to the design effort.

. What should the priorities of the group be -- education, social-emotional support, and/or adherence? The structure of the group will vary, depending on this decision.

If education and skills training are priorities, the sequence of topics should be considered carefully:

. Consider the nature of the chronic condition. What skills would give participants the greatest relief or sense of control? For example, with COPD clients breathing techniques would be a priority.

. Some skills must build on other skills; for example, relaxation must be taught prior to better breathing skills.

. Consider which skills can be performed successfully by participants, given their agility and energy levels. It may be necessary to stage the teaching of a skill across several sessions, with practice inbetween, to ensure that the process will be a rewarding one for the participants.

The decision of whether and how to involve family or friends in the group depends on the group's priorities:

.   Do participants want to discuss personal issues privately, including some which involve family? If yes, it may be better not to invite family, except to selected sessions.

.   Is skills training and adherence help a priority for the group? If yes, it may be useful to have family attend at least once, at intervals, or all of the sessions. They provide the basis for ongoing support after the group has stopped meeting.

.   Do family and clients have a joint need for basic education about the chronic condition and its management? If education is to be the group's priority, consider inviting family to the full sequence of sessions.

Consider environment and mood questions when designing the group:

.   Many participants care about not being labeled as sick or as being part of a "sick" group. The location of the small-group sessions can be one of many subtle cues that reinforces the sick or the health-oriented identity. Consider holding the group at a site away from the health setting, if possible.

.   Another cue is whether leaders wear street clothes instead of "whites."

.   Some small groups purposely schedule a refreshment break immediately following a didactic presentation, to relax the atmosphere and to encourage more informal and personal discussion. Participants can share the responsibility for providing refreshments, again reinforcing an active role.

Group Process

Active participation in the group should be encouraged, as part of motivating active responsibility for care:

.   An introductory statement used for the small groups at the Stanford Arthritis Center is, "We are here to help guide you, but you must ask questions, make decisions, and use a process of trial and error to find what is best for you" (Lorig, 1981).

.   The first session is important for setting a tone of participation. After explaining what you hope the group can address (i.e., the provider's priorities, the reason for the group), consider asking people why they came, what they most want to get from the group. Take a few minutes for people to jot down a few things. Have everyone respond, even if only to say they don't know.

- Encourage questions by indicating that they help everyone in the group learn. Encourage clients to ask any questions they want, and indicate that if the answers aren't available they will be sought for the next meeting.

- Encourage everyone to say something at each session. Reinforce everyone in the group verbally or with a nod.

- Consider the reinforcement effects of different ways of speaking. Leaders may use nonjudgemental verbal reinforcements (e.g., "Thank you") or affirmative ("That's a good point" or "That makes a lot of sense"), or directive ("Did you see how that fits in with what _____ just said?"). The choice and mix of types will depend in part on the priorities, in part on personal style of leaders and participants.

If socio-emotional issues are going to be a priority, the following should be considered:

- The group is likely to benefit from setting a groundrule with respect to confidentiality. One such rule would be to use no names or other obvious identifiers when describing any of the discussion to someone outside the group. A more restrictive rule would be to avoid discussion about the group with anyone not in the group. The dilemma with this latter rule is that at times it may be very helpful for a participant to talk with a family member or friend about an issue which was raised in the group (to describe the viewpoints or experiences of others or put one's own reactions in perspective).

- It is often easiest for participants to start by discussing how they first discovered their condition, early experiences with it, current treatment. Quite a lot of mutual understanding can be established in that fairly neutral territory.

- Since one of the unique opportunities of a peer group is being with others who share one's own experience and perspective, a facilitator should stay "out of the way," staying in the background except to ease a process by which as many people as possible can exchange insights and feelings. It may be that the biggest gift of peer groups is that participants have the opportunity to give to as well as receive from each other.

Continuity across sessions is important, particularly if education or skill building is a priority:

- To encourage continuity across sessions, indicate what the next session will cover. You may wish to suggest that participants work on a specific task between now and the next session, building on material just presented. Examples include recording blood pressure, recording emotional upsets and flare ups, doing an exercise.

. At the beginning of each session, get a debriefing on how things
went during the week. Reinforce participants for their efforts.
It is important to reinforce those who did not follow the regimen,
but who had the courage to return to the next meeting. Encourage a
sense of success rather than failure. Do some problem-solving
around questions that arose from participants' efforts.

If skills training and adherence are both priorities for the
group, the following should be considered in designing the group:

. When skills are taught, a major part of the sessions should be
spent on practice and feedback to participants. It is helpful to
have several leaders so that participants receive adequate
attention and feedback.

. Consider having peers break into pairs to help each other adapt the
principles and skills to their own situation and needs, or to work
out an action plan for applying the principles between now and the
next session.

. Have participants decide how much practice between sessions is
realistic. The goal is to find a level of practice which will
become self-reinforcing.

. If participants are developing their own action plans, at the end
of the session each participant could share it with the larger
group, to get suggestions and to reinforce the commitment to
carrying it out.

. Consider spending time helping participants tailor their regimens
to the constraints of their own situations. Help them identify
specific daily rituals and cues that can remind them to follow the
regimen.

. It is useful to have participants identify social allies who can
help them follow the regimen, or to practice during the week
between meetings. Depending on the goals of the group, it may be
useful to involve these social allies in the meetings themselves.

CLIENT AND STAFF PERSPECTIVES

The small-group literature indicates that participants value their
participation in small groups. As Pavlou (1978) suggests, the group provides
a way for the client to hear information several times, and to hear others
raise questions that he or she might be fearful of asking in a one-on-one
situation with the provider. Conte (1974) reports that participants seemed to
feel a sense of community in being part of a group where having high blood
pressure was the norm. As one participant said, "It's great to be able to say
things with people who understand and to know my feelings are not unique"
(Pavlou and others, 1978). Schwartz and others (1978) describe the example of

one family who became much more able to understand the feelings and physical pain of the participant as a result of hearing others in the group discuss how arthritis affected them. Up to this point, family members had believed that the wife's complaints of pain were exaggerated.

It appears that one of the issues that small groups help participants confront is their fears regarding complications and deterioration. Gross and Brandt (1981) report that participants found themselves much more comfortable with people in worse physical condition than themselves, as a result of their group experience. Pavlou and others (1978) note a similar finding. Clearly, some clients are reluctant to come to a small group. However, once there, these people often have the greatest enthusiasm for both the discussion and practice of the principles presented (Lewis, 1981).

Providers involved in designing and facilitating small groups report enjoying and learning from their involvement. The largest source of satisfaction is from the client's excitement about being with peers and gratitude for learning tangible skills. Likewise, providers report learning more about the context of people's lives, and how regimens must be tailored. Often clients have become quite ingenious and hints for daily living can be gathered from their conversations.

SYSTEM ISSUES

One of the primary issues in doing small groups is the time and cost of advertising and recruiting participants for the group. One suggestion for reducing cost is enlisting the assistance of a local group, such as a voluntary agency, that has experience in promoting health-related programs. Preparation time will be minimized if a basic format can be used again, as new groups are organized. Thus, while two to three hours of preparation may be required for each session the first time that new information or skills are covered, much less preparation time will be required for the same topics in subsequent groups. Some small-group workshop guides are available to build on, which may also reduce preparation time (Lewis, 1981; Lorig and others, 1981).

A second issue is what type of person can lead the groups--specifically, what background or training is needed. While the majority of small group leaders are reported to be health professionals (nurses, physical therapists, psychologists, physicians) an interesting alternative is offered by Lorig (1981). Her small groups are led by a team of two lay people who have gone through a 20-hour training program. A very clear protocol for lay leaders has been developed and is followed for each of the sessions in the small group course. With this direction, leaders are able to function well and keep the cost per person down to $15-20 for the six-week session.

Clearly, the type of training and skills required by group leaders will vary with the priorities of the group. As more emphasis is placed on socio-emotional support and exchange between participants, the more a group leader must have good process skills, particularly the ability to listen well, to focus on client concerns and to involve each participant in the discussion. Even in groups with major emphasis on education and adherence, such process skills will be needed by effective leaders. To help refine some of these skills, Lewis (1981) and Brough (1981) suggest that leader trainees have the opportunity to sit in on a small-group series, to see these skills modeled. Both suggest that a minimum of two days of training would be recommended. As previously stated, Lorig (1981) reports that co-leaders in her groups go through a 20-hour training program.

REFERENCES

Ashikaga, T., and others. Evaluation of a community-based education program for individuals with chronic pulmonary obstructive disease. Journal of Rehabilitation 46:23-27, Apr/Jun 1980.

Brough, K. Personal conversation. Utah Lung Association, Salt Lake City, Utah, August 1981.

Caplan, R. D., and others. Adhering to Medical Regimens: Pilot Experiments in Patient Education and Social Support. Ann Arbor: University of Michigan Press, 1976.

Cole, S. A., and others. Self-help groups for clinic patients with chronic illness. Primary Care 6:325-339, Jun 1979.

Conte, A., and others. Group work with hypertensives. Amer. J. of Nurs. 74:910-912, May 1974.

Dupuis, A., and others. Assessment of the psychological factors and responses in self-managed patients. Diabetes Care 3:117-119, Jan/Feb 1980.

Green, L., and others. Development of randomized patient education experiments with urban poor hypertensives. Patient Counselling and Health Education 1:106-111, Winter-Spring 1977.

Gross, M., and Brandt, K. Educational support groups for patients with ankylosing spondylitis: a preliminary report. Patient Counselling and Health Educ. 3:6-12, First Quarter 1981.

Levine, D., and others. Health education for hypertensive patients. JAMA 241:1700-1703, Apr 1979.

Levine, D., and others. Compliance in hypertension management: what the physician can do. Practical Cardiology 5:151-161, July 1979.

Levy, R. The role of social support in patient compliance: a selective review. In: Haynes, R. B., and others, editors. Patient Compliance to Prescribed Antihypertensive Medication Regimens: A Report to the National Heart, Lung and Blood Institute. Washington: U.S. Department of Health and Human Services, Public Health Service, National Institute of Health, October 1980, 139-164. NIH Publication No. 81-2102.

Lewis, S.O. Building Blocks to Better Breathing. South Burlington, Vermont: American Lung Association of Vermont, 1981.

Lorig, K., and others. A randomized, prospective, controlled study of the effects of health education for people with arthritis. A paper prepared for the American Rheumatism Association Meetings, Boston, Mass., June 1981.

Nessman, D., and others. Increasing compliance in patient-operated hypertension groups. Arch of Internal Med. 140:1427-1430. Nov. 1980. Pavlou, M., and others. Discussion groups for medical patients: a vehicle for improved coping. Psychotherapy and Psychosomatics 30:104-114, 1978.

Pelser, H., and others. Experiences in group discussions with diabetic patients. Psychotherapy and Psychosomatics 32:257-269, 1979.

Peterson, C. M., and Jones, R. L. Feasibility of improved blood glucose control in patients with insulin-dependent diabetes mellitus. Diabetes Care 2:329-335, Jul./Aug. 1979.

Syme, S. Drug treatment of mild hypertension: social and psychological considerations. Annals of New York Acad. of Sciences 99-106, 1978.

Ziesat, H. A. Behavioral modification in the treatment of hypertension. Intern. J. of Psych. in Med. 8:257-265, 2978.

CHAPTER 7
INVOLVEMENT OF FAMILY AND FRIENDS

As Becker and Green (1975) point out, family can strongly influence the commitment and ability of clients to manage their condition. The attitudes and lifestyle of a family can either hinder or aid the client's efforts. The question is how to encourage and focus family cooperation in a way that helps clients manage their condition, and also helps families adjust to living with someone who has a chronic condition.

The literature uses a variety of terms, including "significant other" and "social ally" to refer to close biological and/or emotional relationships which a client has. For simplicity, and to reinforce a broader definition of family, this chapter uses the term "family" to refer both to special friends and immediate family with whom the client lives. Both are assumed to be key sources of support.

Family needs and resources vary widely. Often families want to help a family member, but don't know how. Sometimes, in addition to needing direction, family resentment or fear about the client's condition is paramount. It may become clear, as the provider gathers information about the family's economic and personal circumstances, that the client's condition is the least of the family's worries.

Given a range of situations, it is fortunate that the research on family involvement presents several strategies to use. To help providers choose from among the available strategies, three contexts for involving families will be discussed: 1) home visits, 2) clinic visits, and 3) small groups. For the most part, this research suggests that family involvement can help clients achieve better adherence and health status, particularly when family are given meaningful and specific tasks to do with clients, or when family involvement is combined with other adherence promoting strategies.

HOME VISITS

Several recent studies have examined the impact of home visits on adherence and health status of clients with a chronic condition (Earp and Ory, 1979; Johnson and others, 1978; Katz and others, 1968; Levine and others, 1979; Syme, 1978). Generally, these studies suggest that home visits can improve adherence and health status, particularly for clients known to be at risk for complications or for poor adherence. An important study in this area was conducted with hypertensive clients by Levine and his colleagues (1979). Clients and families received a single home visit in which family members were: 1) told why hypertension needed to be controlled, 2) asked to help the client remember medication and appointments, and 3) asked to identify other ways to help and reinforce the client. At the end of six months, the percentage of clients with controlled blood pressure rose from 37% to 48%. Of the clients at risk for complications from hypertension, 22% brought their blood pressure down to the goal, compared to 11% of the clients believed to be at lower risk (Morisky, 1980).

A similar finding is suggested by a second study involving both self-monitoring of blood pressure and monthly home visits (Johnson and others, 1978). Unlike the Levine study, however, no special effort was made to involve family. For clients who expected to have trouble remembering to take their medications, the home visits and self-monitoring had a positive impact on blood pressure control; but this was not true for other clients. The two findings together suggest that it may be useful to target the more costly interventions such as home visits for those clients who have been identified as being at risk because they have more complex regimens, expect to have trouble remembering or coping with the regimen, or are known to be at risk for complications.

Home visits affect the provider as well as the client and family. When a provider steps into the client's home, it is much more likely that he or she can develop a realistic sense of the client's resources for managing a regimen (Katz and others, 1968). A number of researchers have indicated that during home visits family are likely to discuss problems that are not directly related to the client's condition--financial problems, for example, or concerns about a teenager in the family (Earp and Ory, 1979; Syme, 1978). In the process, the provider develops a better perspective on how the regimen and condition fit into the family's life. This perspective then contributes to the process of staff and client mutually designing a regimen that is realistic for the client and family.

SMALL GROUPS

A second means of involving family is provided through small groups. As discussed in the preceding chapter, family members are often invited to attend small group sessions (Ashikaga and others, 1980; Gross and Brandt, 1981; Lorig, 1981; Schwartz and others, 1978). However, it is rare that small groups identify specific ways that families can help the client manage his or her condition. Some weight loss studies suggest an inexpensive model for doing this.

Participants in two small group studies on weight loss asked a person of their choice to attend one of their group sessions. In one study this person served as a witness while the participant signed a behavioral contract designed during a small group session (Ureda, 1980). Subsequently, the witness attended a small group meeting where each contract commitment was reviewed. Participants whose behavioral contracts were witnessed, lost weight significantly faster than did group participants without a witness. In the second study, family were divided into two groups. During a single group session, the first group of family learned how to reinforce the client's weight loss (i.e., pounds lost), while the second group learned how to reinforce the clients appropriate eating behavior (e.g., not snacking) (Saccone and Israel, 1978). In this second study the group who was reinforced for appropriate eating behavior lost twice as much weight (13 pounds) as did the participants reinforced for weight loss. The control group of nonparticipants gained four pounds during the two-month period. Thus, both studies indicate that a single small group session can be used to focus the attention of family on the behavioral commitments made by the participant.

This finding is consistent with the Steckel and Swain work (1977; 1981), which also emphasizes the importance of identifying specific do-able behaviors whose achievement can be reinforced during a clinic visit.

CLINIC VISITS

Clinic visits represent a third way to involve family in the client's attempts to manage a chronic condition. One difficulty in evaluating this option is that relatively little research examines how to involve families during clinic visits. Family involvement seems to increase client adherence most when family are taught a specific and meaningful task, such as blood pressure measurement (Baranowski and others, 1978). Without this specific focus,. family involvement appears to have less effect on adherence (Glanz and others, 1981). Neither study evaluated the emotional benefits for family and/or client of having family attend a clinic visit. Given the absence of more research on what should transpire during the visit, the small group findings on weight loss and contracting will be applied to suggest one type of interaction that may be effective.

The weight loss and contracting research suggests that focusing attention on client behaviors helps lead to the achievement of health goals. This literature also suggests it is useful for significant others to reinforce specific behaviors which the client had contracted to do (Ureda, 1980; Saccone and Israel, 1978). Applying this to clinic visits, one way to involve family would be for clients to define specific behaviors which they want help doing, identify ways that significant others can aid or reinforce clients for performing these behaviors, and help significant others clarify how realistic it would be to do what is being negotiated. This model suggests that in essence the significant other is developing a verbal contract to help the client in a specific way. Future research may more fully evaluate this and other approaches for involving family during clinic visits.

KEY COMPONENTS

The research just reviewed suggests that under certain circumstances family involvement can help clients manage their regimens, particularly when family are given meaningful, specific tasks that mesh with the client's priorities. This research is still at an early phase, but the findings, combined with recommendations from providers who work with families, suggest the following key issues to consider when involving families.

ASSESSMENT ISSUES

. Does the client want to involve any family? If yes, have the client select who would be most helpful, in terms of the supportive nature of the person, and the frequency of contact.

. Is now a good time for the family member or significant other to become involved? At times family will be absorbed in other economic and personal concerns which may make it difficult to give good attention to the chronic condition. If this is the case, consider referrals which may help the family deal with these and focus their attention on only a few issues concerning the client's condition. If family or friends are reluctant to play a more involved role, reassure them that general support for the client in his or her efforts is significant in and of itself.

. In deciding how extensively to involve assess the following:

  - Does the client expect to have trouble remembering medications or adhering to regimens?

  - Does the client have a complex regimen?

  - Is the client known to be at risk of complications?

  - Does the client have a history of nonadherence?

. If any of the above are true, consider involving family more aggressively than just through education and ongoing contact with staff (which should be offered to all families).

METHOD FOR INVOLVEMENT

Methods for involving family members in adherence include the following:

. If home visits are made, take advantage of the opportunity to assess other sources of stress in the family, apart from the chronic condition. This may provide the most helpful information for realistically adapting the health goals and regimen to fit the client and family resources.

. Make sure that the client and family understand the benefits of the recommended regimen and that there is an opportunity for both to raise any questions or special concerns they have about the regimen or condition. Make sure also that both client and family member are comfortable with the role suggested for the family member.

. Consider identifying an action plan for the family member to assist the client, one which the client believes would be helpful and which the family member feels would be realistic. The action plan can identify specific behaviors for the client and family members.

. Try to identify tangible tasks, such as blood pressure measurement, that family can do and that the client agrees would be helpful.

. If family is to be involved via clinic visits, make sure the receptionist is alerted to schedule appointments at a time that is convenient for the chosen family member as well as the client.

. If small groups are to be used, consider having a person selected
by the client attend at least one session. At this session each
participant's behavioral contract or action plan can be reviewed.
Also, the group can clarify the specific role of the chosen person
in reinforcing and aiding the client's self-management efforts, for
example in supporting concrete eating, exercise, medication-taking
behaviors of the client.

CLIENT AND PROVIDER PERSPECTIVES

In a series of interviews conducted with individuals who had hypertension,
clients reported that they understood hypertension and in general knew how it
was to be managed, but were confused about the specifics of their own
regimens. They also reported a need for family encouragement to control high
blood pressure (Green and others, 1979). Family support thus appears to be a
critical variable.

Research by Glanz and others (1981) provide more specific information on
client perspective of family involvement through clinic visits. A nurse met
with clients who had hypertension and with a person of their choice. Sixty
percent considered the meeting useful and 57% found it reassuring. Almost all
(94.7%) said that their person of choice helped with the regimen.

Earp and Ory (1979) in their research on family involvement through home
visits and blood pressure measurement of clients reports that the visiting
nurses felt the family involvement was valuable. Nurses were able to
understand how the client's condition fit into the rest of the family's
priorities. Given that many of the families had considerable economic and
personal problems, it was easier to understand how the client's self
management efforts needed to be tailored further.

SYSTEM ISSUES

This chapter discussed three strategies for involving family in clients'
attempts to manage their condition. Some of the strategies, such as home
visits, are clearly more costly than others, and therefore it is useful to
discuss suggestions for minimizing these costs.

Home visits represent a potentially powerful intervention for family
involvement and an excellent data source for providers. Unfortunately, it is
prohibitively expensive in most outpatient settings for staff to visit all
clients who have chronic conditions. Two approaches to reduce the costs of
this strategy might be considered. Research on home visits suggests that
public health nurses can perform a home visit function quite effectively,
particularly if good coordination exists with the primary care provider (Katz
and others, 1968; Earp and Ory, 1979). This approach minimizes cost to the
primary health care provider by requiring only that a good reporting system be
established between two points in the health care system.

A second approach for primary care staff to consider is targeting selected individuals to receive the more costly home visit intervention. Specifically, staff might choose the following clients to consider for a home visit: those known to be at risk of complications, those who have complex regimens, those with a history of nonadherence, those who expect to have problems with the regimen, and those who request a home visit.

Further, it may be useful to devise a stepped approach for this target group of clients. McClellan and others (1980) describe a program in which hypertensive clients are seen every two weeks until their blood pressure is controlled. If a client does not respond to the follow-up, then a home visit is made. Thus, home visits could be viewed as the third phase of a protocol developed specifically to help clients at risk for complications and/or nonadherence.

Small groups represent another possibility for involving family effectively. The primary costs associated with small groups have been discussed in their own chapter and will not be discussed in length here. However, involving the family implies very little additional cost over the basic expense of running group sessions for clients. From the weight reduction literature, it appears that even a single session involvement of family can be beneficial.

Clinic visits represent the third strategy for involving family. If, as Baranowski and others (1980) suggest, providers use the visit to teach families a specific skill such as blood pressure control, lengthier visits will need to be scheduled. This would also be true if action plans were to be negotiated with clients and families. To help receptionists schedule 30 minute visits, it is useful to scan the entire week for regular times when longer visits can be managed. If a nurse is doing the primary education with families, she or he may wish to reserve some regular spots when more time and exam room space is available. An example of such a time may be when a team physician is away from the clinic or office setting, perhaps during hospital rounds. If providers other than physicians are doing this teaching it will be important to establish protocols for the education and negotiation with family which are consistent with the setting's practice. Therefore, staff time will be needed to review the protocol before it is used. Periodic staff meetings are useful to keep team members informed of the outcomes and any problems with the protocol.

REFERENCES

Ashikaga, T., and others. Evaluation of a community-based education program for individuals with chronic pulmonary obstructive disease. J. of Rehabil. 46:23-27, Apr/Jun 1980.

Baranowski, T., and others. A rural mining community high blood pressure control project. A paper presented at a poster session of the National Conference on High Blood Pressure Control, Los Angeles, California, April 3, 1978. p 4.

Baranowski, T., and others. Utilization and medication compliance for high blood pressure: an experiment with family involvement and self blood pressure monitoring in a rural population, Amer. J. of Rural Health, 6:51-67, 1980.

Becker, M., and Green, L. A family approach to compliance with medical treatment: a selective review of the literature. Int. J. of Health Educ. 18:173-182, Mar 1975.

Earp, J., and Ory, M. G. The effects of social support and health professional home visits on patient adherence to hypertension regimens. A paper presented at the National Conference on High Blood Pressure Control, Washington, D.C., April 6, 1979.

Glanz, K., and others. Initial knowledge and attitudes as predictors of intervention effects: the individual management plan. Patient Counselling and Health Educ. 3:30-42, First Quarter 1981.

Glanz, K., and others. Linking research and practice in patient education for hypertension patient responses to four educational interventions. Med. Care 19:141-152, Feb 1981.

Green, L., and others. Development of randomized patient education experiments with urban poor hypertensives. Patient Counselling and Health Educ. 1:106-111, 1979.

Gross, M., and Brandt, K. Educational support groups for patients with ankylosing spondylitis: a preliminary report. Patient Counselling and Health Educ. 3:6-12, First Quarter 1981.

Johnson, A., and others. Self-recording of blood pressure in the management of hypertension. Can. Med. Assoc. J. 119:1034-1039, Nov 4, 1978.

Katz, S., and others. Comprehensive outpatient care in rheumatoid arthritis. JAMA 206:1249-1254, Nov 4, 1968.

Levine, D., and others. Health education for hypertensive patients. JAMA 241:1700-1703, Apr 1979.

Levine, D., and others. Compliance in hypertension management: What the physician can do. Practical Cardiology 5:151-161, Jul 1979.

Lorig, K., and others. A randomized, prospective, controlled study of the effects of health education for people with Arthritis. A paper prepared for the American Rheumatism Association Meetings, Boston, Mass., Jun 1981.

McClellan, W., and others. Prolonged blood pressure control in a rural outpatient hypertension clinic: a description of methodology and results. Presented at National Conference on High Blood Pressure Control, Los Angeles, 1978.

Morisky, D., and others. The relative impact of health education for low- and high-risk patients with hypertension. Preventive Med. 9:550-558, Jul 1980.

Nessman, D., and others. Increasing compliance in patient-operated hypertension groups. Arch. of Intern. Med. 140:1427-1430, Nov 1980.

Pavlou, M., and others. Discussion groups for medical patients: a vehicle for improved coping. Psychotherapy and Psychosomatics 30:104-114, 1978.

Pelser, H., and others. Experiences in group discussions with diabetic patients. Psychotherapy and Psychosomatics 32:257-269, 1979.

Peterson, C. M., and Jones, R. L. Feasibility of improved blood glucose control in patients with insulin-dependent diabetes mellitus. Diabetes Care 2:329-335, Jul/Aug 1979.

Saccone, A., and Israel, A. Effects of experimenter versus significant other controlled reinforcement and choice of target behavior on weight loss. Behavior Therapy 9:271-278, Mar 1978.

Schwartz, L., and others. Multidisciplinary group therapy for rheumatoid arthritis, Psychosomatics 19(5):289-293, May 1978.

Steckel, S. B. Increasing adherence of outpatients to therapeutic regimens. Project Final Report. Ann Arbor: Veterans Administration, Health Services Research and Development Project #343, 1981.

Steckel, S. B., and Swain, M. A. Contracting with patients to improve compliance. Hospitals 51:81-84, 1977.

Swain, M. A., and Steckel, S. B. Influencing adherence among hypertensives. Research in Nursing and Health 4:213-222, Mar 1981.

Syme, S. Drug treatment of mild hypertension: social and psychological considerations. Annual of New York Academy of Sciences 99-106, 1978.

Ureda, J. R. The effect of contract witnessing on motivation and weight loss in a weight control program. Health Education Quarterly 7(3):163-185, Fall 1980.

Wyka, C. A., and others. Group education for the hypertensive. Cardiovascular Nursing 16:1-5, Jan/Feb 1980.

Ziesat, H. A. Behavioral modification in the treatment of hypertension. Int. J. of Psychiat. in Med. 8:257-265, 1977-1978.

CHAPTER 8
SYSTEMS SUPPORT STRATEGIES

MAIL AND TELEPHONE CONTACT

As Katz and others (1968) point out, management of a chronic condition is not a rigid set of behaviors following a single set of goals worked out in a clinic or office. Good management is a dynamic process of changing goals and regimens, based on the client's experience. If staff are to help clients refine and adhere to their ongoing management plans, it is necessary to keep a relationship with clients for followup. The following section discusses postcard and telephone contact with clients as two cost-effective ways of encouraging clients to remain in care, in order to adapt regimens and treatment goals to the client's changing needs.

Positive results have been reported for both phone and mail follow-up. Studies have consistently found that using mailed appointment reminders can decrease missed appointments for clients with chronic or acute conditions (Go and Becker, 1979; Schroeder, 1973; Takala and others, 1979). In one of the most complete studies in this area, Schroeder (1973) examined three different approaches to remind clients of their appointments: 1) Five days before their scheduled appointment 125 clients were sent a postcard reminder; 2) The day before the visit 125 other clients were telephoned by the team nurse to remind them of the appointment; 3) A staff physician made the reminder phone call to another 125 clients, also the day before the visit. A control group of 125 clients received no reminders. The group of clients who received the postcard had the lowest missed appointment rate (13.9%). For clients receiving the physician call it was 17.6%; for clients receiving the nurse call it was 19.5%. Clients receiving no reminder had a missed rate of 24.6%.

At first it may seem surprising that the phone call didn't result in better appointment-keeping rates. However, 42% of clients to be telephoned were never reached. Those who were reached by phone had a missed rate of only 12%, still only slightly lower than the postcard rate. The authors conclude that postcards are the most effective way of substantially reducing broken appointment rates. Similar findings are reported by Go and Becker (1979), who showed that contacting clients by postcard 1-2 days prior to their appointments is far more effective than calling them immediately following a missed appointment. The missed rates of clients who were contacted immediately after an appointment continued to be as high as clients not contacted, whereas clients contacted 1-2 days prior to an appointment showed considerable improvement in appointment keeping.

Given that clinic resources are often limited, a key question is whether staff can target certain clients to receive postcards. There is some indication that health care settings can predict the client groups most needing postcard follow-up. In recent research by Dove and Schneider (1981) four characteristics were found to predict the pattern of broken appointments. The strongest predictor of whether a client breaks appointments in the future is whether he or she has broken them in the past. Another important variable is the interval between appointments. Nineteen per cent of appointments were broken when they were less than six weeks apart versus 28% broken when they were more than six weeks apart. Younger age and greater distance from the clinic were also predictors of missed appointments. Thus it may be that the appointment reminder card system can go into effect at the point when a client misses an appointment and/or has a combination of the above characteristics.

Mail and phone follow-up have also been studied as a means for promoting adherence to self management regimens. Takala and others (1979), in a study of 200 people with hypertension in Finland, used follow-up postcards to remind clients of their next visit and also to indicate what their blood pressure had been and what medications were prescribed during the visit. Only 4% of the group receiving postcards dropped out of the treatment, as compared to 19% of a group of clients without the follow-up card. Further, of those who stayed in treatment, 94% in the postcard group but only 78% of the control group reduced their blood pressure by at least 10% over a one year period.

In a brief study with diabetic clients, Etzwiler (1980), used phone calls with a group of clients who had signed contracts. The phone calls encouraged clients to test and record their urine values over a two week period. Results showed that the phone calls increased adherence from 52% to 64% when staff called clients once, and to 80% when staff called twice. Since the study was limited in design and length, findings should be viewed accordingly; but they do suggest that phone calls deserve to be examined further as a tool to achieve adherence.

As further evidence of the potential of phone calls, Bertera and Bertera (1981) examined the effect of using five-minute phone conversations in follow-up counseling with hypertensive clients. The client population was predominantly Black, elderly, female, and poor. For six months 20 clients received counseling and reinforcement for weight control, sodium restriction, medication adherence, appointment keeping, and coping with personal or family relationship problems. Half were counseled by a social worker every 3 weeks by phone, while the others were counseled during clinic visits, also at 3 week intervals. A control group of 20 clients randomly drawn from clinic records received only their routine care. Over a six-month period, the blood pressure of both the clinic counseling and telephone counseling groups decreased significantly while the blood pressure of clients receiving routine care rose slightly. Results indicate that nearly 90% of all telephone counseling contacts were completed as planned; because of missed appointments, only 63% of the clinic visit sessions were attended as scheduled. Thus, this study, more than others, clarifies that phone contact has clear potential for augmenting clinic counseling visits.

Key Components

The literature suggests a number of dimensions to consider when deciding to use reminder postcards or phone calls:

. If the purpose of the communication is solely to decrease broken appointments, postcard reminders are more cost-effective than the phone calls.

. Reminder cards are most effective if received 1-2 days prior to an appointment. Contacting a client immediately <u>after</u> a broken appointment is generally ineffective.

. Cards should include the appointment time and a number to call if the client wishes to cancel and reschedule. An option is to include on the card the medication and blood pressure readings (or other health status measures) from earlier visits.

. If staff wish to target the postcards solely at clients most likely to break appointments and drop out of care, the best predictor is the past record of missed appointments. After a client misses an appointment, reminder cards can be sent just prior to the next scheduled visit. This is particularly helpful if visits are more than a month apart.

. Phone calls can be cost effective if more than an appointment reminder is intended. For example, calls can be useful for counseling or adherence support.

. If phone contact is done, staff should establish protocols for the type of information and questions that the caller is to address with the client over the phone.

. It is important to ask clients whether they would like to have follow-up by phone. Some clients will prefer this option over any other. Many elderly or relatively homebound persons will prefer the phone, if there is not much difficulty with hearing or with mobility to get to the phone. To minimize time lost on unanswered calls, negotiate a range of times that would be convenient for the calls to be received.

Client/Provider Perspectives

The most common reasons clients give for broken appointments is that they forgot or misunderstood the time (41.5%); had health, money, or family problems (19%); or had a schedule conflict (12.8%) (Go and Becker, 1979). Client response to card and phone calls from staff is generally positive, although the calls make more impact on some clients than on others. In interviews with clients who received a single phone call from a nurse to reinforce their adherence, Glanz and others (1981) report that 33% did not remember receiving the phone call.

Interviews with clients who receive phone calls from providers suggest that often clients are grateful for providers' efforts and a telephone call is interpreted by some as an extra sign of caring. Providers who use telephone contact report that they find phone calls with clients useful, particularly if the provider has a scheduled time to make and receive calls. Many client concerns can be handled relatively easily over the phone. Thus, the phone call augments, rather than replaces, the normal client visit.

System Issues

With respect to postcards, some physicians report reluctance to mail
appointment reminders for fear it seems like advertising. This is an
interesting contrast to the dental profession, which has long used mail
reminders. Postcards are more cost-effective than telephone calls for
reminding clients about their scheduled clinic appointments. Oppenheim and
others (1979) indicate that a volunteer or receptionist requires 1 1/2 minutes
per appointment for postcards, but 4 1/2 minutes per appointment for a single
telephone call. This may be a low estimate for phone call time, since often
more than a single call is necessary to reach the client. As Schroeder (1973)
found, as many as 42% of the clients were not reached by phone because they
were out.

The cost of phone calls as reminders may be higher than mail contact;
however, phone calls do provide the opportunity to follow-up on regimens, and
to provide additional counseling and problem-solving assistance. If the phone
is being used for the purpose of counseling clients the cost is more
appropriately compared to the cost of a clinic visit rather than a postcard.
When phone costs are compared in this fashion the cost per client with
controlled hypertension over a six month period was found to be $82.00 for a
clinic visit every three weeks versus $39.00 for telephone counseling every
three weeks (Bertera and Bertera, 1981). It appears that phone contact does
have potential as a cost-effective strategy for helping clients to manage a
chronic condition.

REFERENCES

Bertera, E., and Bertera, R. The cost-effectiveness of telephone versus
clinic counseling for hypertensive patients: A pilot study. Amer. J. of
Public Health 71(6):626-627, Jun 1981.

Dove, H. G., and Schneider, K. C. The usefulness of patients' individual
characteristics in predicting no-shows in outpatient clinics. Med. Care
19:734-740, Jul 1981.

Etzwiller, D. D., Teaching allied health professionals about self-management.
Diabetes Care 3(1):121-123, Jan 1980.

Glanz, K., and others. Initial knowledge and attitudes as predictors of
intervention effects: the individual management plan. Patient Counselling
and Health Educ. 3:30-42, First Quarter 1981.

Go, H., and Becker, H. Reducing broken appointments in a primary care
clinic. J. of Ambulatory Care Manage. 23-30, May 1979.

Katz, S., and others. Comprehensive outpatient care in rheumatoid arthritis.
JAMA 206(6):1249-1254, Nov 4, 1968.

Oppenheim, G. L., and others. Failed appointments: a review. J. of Family
Practice 8(4):789-796, 1979.

Schroeder, S. Lowering broken appointment rates at a medical clinic.
<u>Med. Care</u> 11:75-78, Jan-Feb 1973.

Takala, J., and others. Improving compliance with therapeutic regimens in
hypertensive patients in a community health center. <u>Circulation</u>
59(3):540-543, Mar 1979.

CHAPTER 9
CONCLUSION

The self management strategies described in this book have effects beyond promoting adherence. Before selecting a strategy, providers will want to consider the client's total profile of health and socio-emotional needs. For example, one client may be socially isolated and gain multiple benefits from attending a group on self-management. Another client may be struggling with a lost sense of control that self-blood pressure measurement or medical record co-authoring might help. As suggested in Chapter 1, the selection of strategies will be assisted by developing a step approach protocol for the client population, however the need for provider judgement based on the individual client profile still exists.

The fact that strategies have multiple effects is beneficial for the provider as well as the client. Self-management strategies may assist providers in operationalizing the type of client-provider process they value. The research field for adherence is still at an early stage, and it is unclear how several self-management strategies have their impact. However, one hypothesis is that adherence strategies basically formalize critical elements of an effective client-provider relationship. For example, it may be that a strategy such as contracting helps providers to clearly address the client's agenda, develop realistic action plans tailored to the client's daily life, follow up on the client's concerns and action plan at each visit, and adjust regimens as client priorities and self-awareness change. In reality the client-provider relationship is as important as the strategies used to promote self-management. As Schulman (1979) points out, some of these strategies may help providers ensure that all of their clients receive consistent follow-up and support.

Ultimately, the question of what is a quality client-provider relationship is an ongoing personal question which providers address throughout their careers. Different providers will arrive at different definitions. As readers experiment with strategies offered in this book, personal definitions are likely to continue to be refined. It is hoped that readers will use this book as one more of many stimuli for this ongoing process of self-reflection. As one last offering to this effort, this book ends with a client's personal definition of a client-provider relationship which has been very important in her efforts to regulate diabetes:

"I have a doctor now who takes the time and just listens and takes in what I say and works with it. He doesn't listen to it and try to say, 'what is she really asking' He just works with what I say....He tries to fit my diabetes care to my lifestyle rather than fit my lifestyle to my diabetes, because he knows I wouldn't do that anyway. He works on a problem until it is solved. He'll say, 'we'll keep working on it until we get it. We're not going to give up.'...He does a lot to help me problem solve; handle problems at home....I have a real sense of friendship and openness...just that he really cares, and that's very important to me."

GLOSSARY

Control Group

A control group serves as a comparison for another group being studied. Usually the control group receives routine care, and the other group receives some special teaching or training. For example, two groups may be compared to see what effect contracting has on blood pressure. In this case, the group that receives routine care, but no contracts, serves as a control group.

Intervention or Treatment

The special teaching, training, or support offered to try to improve client care, knowledge, attitudes, behavior or physical health.

Experimental Group

People are assigned to different study groups; i.e., either a control or experimental group. Experimental (often called treatment) groups get the special intervention being studied; for example, contracting, group educational classes, or home care.

Random Assignment

Assignment of clients to control or experimental groups is done in such a way that people have an equal chance of being chosen for either group. This minimizes the likelihood that the groups will be different because of attitudes, experiences or personal characteristics and helps ensure that any differences in the impact of the treatment intervention can be attributed to the intervention rather than to differences between people in the two groups.

Demographics

As used here demographics refers to things like the age, gender, educational or income level, or race of the population being studied. If the clients being studied are demographically different from your client population, the same intervention with your clients may not yield the same results.

Limitations of Inference

Any aspects of the study that suggest one should be careful about drawing conclusions or generalizing from the study's results.

Pre- and Post-Measures

A measure of client's attitude, knowledge, behavior skill, or physical condition before (pre-) and after (post-) an intervention like contracting. The two measures can be compared to help determine if the intervention had any impact on the client (for example, blood pressure might change for clients participating in contracting).

Sometimes a post-measurement alone is done; for example, if a client is newly diagnosed with a chronic condition that requires routine administration of medications, it may not be possible to collect preintervention measures of the client's ability to adhere to recommended medication regimens.

Reliability of the Instrument	An instrument (test, questionnaire, interview protocol) is reliable when it consistently yields the same assessment of the same thing (i.e., a client's attitude, behavior or knowledge). For example, a questionnaire or test might be divided in half so that clients are asked 1/2 of the questions one day and 1/2 of the questions the next day. If both parts of the questionnaire yield the same assessment of what is being measured, the instrument would be reliable.
Validity of the Instrument	A measurement tool like a questionnaire or test is valid if it measures the content it is meant to measure. For example, if clients are asked questions about their adherence, the questions must be carefully worded or the questionnaire may only measure the client's desire to please the interviewer by responding positively or to avoid embarrassment.
Sample Size	Sample size is a statistical term that means the number of clients being studied. The number of clients in both the control and experimental groups must be large enough to allow the use of statistics to help determine if any change in client behaviors, attitudes, or physical condition occurs because of the intervention rather than by chance.

ANNNOTATED BIBLIOGRAPHY

Following is an annotated bibliography of several references, cited in earlier chapters. It was anticipated that some readers would want to examine studies in more detail than was possible in the text of the preceding chapters. Because much of the adherence research literature has serious methodological problems, only a subgroup of adherence studies have been included. Criteria for including references were that the studies:

1)   focus on individuals being treated on an out-patient basis for arthritis, COPD, diabetes, or hypertension;

2)   examine a strategy to promote self-management;

3)   use an outcome measure relevant for adherence; and

4)   either meet accepted research standards (control groups, client sample size, reliable outcome measures) or provide particularly interesting qualitative information about the client-provider experience.

To aid providers in the task of reading this literature critically, the bibliography describes each study in terms of the client population, purpose of the study, design of the study, interventions or strategies used with clients, outcome measures, results, and limitations of inference common to studies of this type. A glossary of terms, used to discuss common limitations of inference, precedes the annotated bibliography.

The annotations have been indexed in the Topical Guide to Annotated References to assist readers in finding citations most relevant to their practice. References are numbered according to the order they appear in the bibliography (which is alphabetical). For example, number 1 in the Guide refers to the first reference listed in the bibliography, "Ashikaga and others."

The upper half of the Guide indexes the references by the type of self-management strategy the study used with clients. Readers interested in starting small groups can turn to the list of references which document the use of small groups, while other readers interested in other strategies, such as telephone or postcard contact, can quickly turn to these categories. In the lower half of the table, references are categorized by the outcome measures used in the described studies. Readers interested in increasing medication adherence can examine references which specifically describe studies that assessed either medication adherence, or health status measures such as blood pressure. It is hoped this Guide will ease the task of locating references most relevant to the individual reader's needs.

TOPICAL GUIDE TO ANNOTATED REFERENCES

	DIABETES	HYPERTENSION	COPD	ARTHRITIS	OTHER CONDITIONS
ADHERENCE/SELF-MANAGEMENT STRATEGIES					
Contracting/ Medical Record Co-authoring	8, 9, 26	24, 25, 26, 9		26	13, 14, 24, 29
Self-Monitoring	6, 8, 15 22	2, 7, 10, 12, 16, 20, 21			23
Small Group	6, 15, 22	4, 17, 19, 20, 27, 30, 31, 32	1	18	29
Family Involvement		2, 7, 10, 16, 17, 19, 31, 32			23
Postcard/Telephone	8	3, 10, 28			(5) 11
ADHERENCE MEASURES					
Medication Adherence		2, 4, 10, 12, 16, 17, 19, 20, 21, 24, 30	1	18	
Exercise	22	31	1	18	14
Health Status (e.g., blood (pressure)	6, 15, 22 26	2, 3, 4, 7, 12, 16, 17, 19, 20, 21, 24, 25, 26, 27, 28, 30, 31, 32		26	13, 14, 23 29
Diet	26	2, 10, 17, 19, 21, 26			23
Appointment Keeping	9, 26	9, 17, 20 25, 26, 30		26	5, 11

Numbers 1, 2, 3, etc. refer to alphabetical listing of attached annotated references.

1. ASHIKAGA, T., and others. Evaluation of a community-based education program for individuals with chronic pulmonary obstructive disease. Journal of Rehabilitation 46:23-27, Apr-Jun 1980.

>Population Studied: 64 volunteers, clients with COPD, mostly male, aged 37-82.

>Purpose: To evaluate a workshop program designed to assist individuals in knowledge, motivation, and psychological support.

>Design: 4 month study; random assignment of volunteers; 1 control, 1 experimental group; pre- and post-treatment tests.

>Interventions: Workshop participants in May constituted the treatment group, the control group was composed of clients on a waiting list for the September group. Breathing workshops consisted of six 2-hour sessions attended by clients and family members. They covered medication, complications, nutrition, effective coughing, breathing retraining, relaxation and mobility exercises, building physical endurance, and basic respiratory anatomy and physiology. Small group discussion was included, to aid participants in identifying and coping with problems arising from living with COPD. Participants learned and practiced skills in the first hour of each session. Group discussion followed in the second hour.

>Measures: (a) Understanding and knowledge of COPD, (b) adherence to self-help activities, (c) readiness to take action, (d) affect.

>Results: Persons in the treatment group had significant increases in their knowledge of COPD performance of self-help activities and readiness to take action. Surprisingly, nonparticipants' perceived social disability decreased more and their perceived chance of improvement increased more than was true for participants.

>Limitations of Inference: The volunteer sample, predominantly males, suggests the need for a broader sample in future studies. The authors suggest that it would be useful to validate self-report with more objective measures of adherence.

2. BARANOWSKI, T., and others. Utilization and medication compliance for high blood pressure: An experiment with family involvement and self blood pressure monitoring in a rural population. American Journal of Rural Health 6(1-6):51-67, 1980.

Population Studied: 126 hypertensives from 2 sources--1 group
previously undetected, predominantly male, most less than 9th
grade education, and screened at a mine site; the 2nd group
referred to the nurse hypertension counselor from other
providers at the clinic.

Purpose: To test an intervention that anticipated and addressed
potential sources of nonadherence.

Design: Duration not stated; random assignment; 1 control and 3
experimental groups; pre- and post-measures.

Interventions: (a) Control group received no special
intervention. (b) 1st experimental group: clients were taught
self-monitoring of their own blood pressure. (c) 2nd group:
clients were asked to bring along a "significant other," at
first to each clinic visit, then to every other visit. This
ally was encouraged to help the clinic adhere by problem
solving, taking blood pressure, and reinforcing behaviors. (d)
3rd group: both interventions.

Measures: (a) Blood pressure; (b) medication adherence; (c)
low-sodium diet adherence.

Results: (a) Diastolic blood pressure control was achieved by
clients receiving both interventions, and by the control group,
receiving neither. Controlled diastolic blood pressure was not
achieved by clients receiving either blood pressure
self-monitoring or family involvement alone. (b) There were no
significant differences in medication adherence across the
groups; 90% reported taking all or most of their medications.
(c) There were no significant differences in reported salt
consumption between groups.

Limitations of Inference: A predominantly male sample was
used. Adherence was quite high across all groups (90%) so it
would have been difficult to see improvement. The group
receiving neither blood pressure self-monitoring nor family
involvement was still part of an aggressive treatment program
which included contracting, medication self-monitoring forms,
and phone call reminders (provided to all clients in care). The
aggressiveness of this program appears to have contributed to
the positive findings for the control group.

3. BERTERA, E. M., and Bertera, R. L. The cost-effectiveness of
    telephone versus clinic counseling for hypertensive patients: a
    pilot study. American Journal of Public Health 71(6):626-627, Jun
    1981.

    Population Studied: 40 clients with hypertension; outpatient;
    predominantly Black, elderly, female, and poor.

Purpose: To test whether telephone counseling is as effective and cost-effective as face-to-face counseling for hypertensive clients.

Design: 6-month study; matched sample (not random): 1 control (20) and 2 experimental groups (10 each); pre- and post-measures.

Interventions: (a) All clients received routine medical care. (b) 1st experimental group clients were also counseled by phone every 3 weeks. All counseling contacts covered medication, weight control, sodium restriction. (c) 2nd experimental group clients received individual counseling on the same topics but face-to-face at the clinic.

Measures: (a) Blood pressure (BP); (b) cost.

Results: (a) Median blood pressure in the telephone and clinic counseling groups declined significantly; the control group remained unchanged. (b) The cost per client with diastolic blood pressure under control was $82 for the clinic counseling and $39 for the telephone counseling strategy.

Limitations of Inference: Small sample; no random assignment from a large pool of eligible hypertensives; this should be considered a pilot study. Although telephone counseling was effective with this lower income, elderly female client sample, it would be useful to test its effectiveness with other general population groups.

4. CAPLAN, R. D., and others. Adhering to Medical Regimens: Pilot Experiments in Patient Education and Social Support. Ann Arbor: University of Michigan Press, 1976.

Population Studied: 200 ambulatory clients with hypertension.

Purpose: To develop interventions for increasing client adherence and to test underlying hypotheses about social support and other potential determinants of adherence.

Design: 1 year; random assignment; 1 control group and 2 experimental groups; pre- and post-test.

Interventions: (a) All clients received routine care. (b) One experimental group also attended a series of 4 weekly 1-hour lectures on the nature of high blood pressure and its treatment. (c) The other experimental group (social support group) clients attended a series of 6 2-hour weekly classes run by a trained nurse clinician, covering same information as in the lecture group, but also providing social-emotional support through various discussion techniques and role plays dealing with adherence behavior.

Measures: (a) Blood pressure (BP); (b) adherence to regimens.

Results: (a) 3 types of variables were associated with levels of BP--self-reported adherence, accurate knowledge of their regimens, perception of consequences of nonadherence as serious; (b) there was relative gain in information about health care between pre- and post-tests, a relative increase in reported ability to take care of one's own health, higher motivation to adhere, more serious attitudes about the health consequences of nonadherence, and greater levels of self-reported adherence. There were no differences in the amount of change of BP levels among the 3 groups for the interval between the pre- and post-test sample, although the sample as a whole showed a significant drop in blood pressure levels.

Limitations of Inference: Only preliminary data is reported. Authors note that similarity in content between lecture and social support group blurred the contrast.

5. DOVE, H. G., and Schneider, K. C. The usefulness of patients' individual characteristics in predicting no-shows in outpatient clinics. Medical Care 19:734-740, Jul 1981.

Population Studied: 756 clients with scheduled appointments at an eastern VA Medical Center.

Purpose: To develop a model to predict which clients will keep their appointments, based on individual client characteristics.

Design: A predictive model based on one sample of 179 medical records was tested on a second sample of 577 medical records.

Analysis Used to Create Predictive Model: A number of variables were abstracted from the medical records, such as race, age, type of visit, appointment interval, and previous appointment-keeping record. Analysis tested the association between each of these variables and the dependent variable "extent of appointment breaking." Based on this, a model predicting client appointment-keeping behavior was developed and tested using another group of clients at the same setting.

Results: (a) The strongest variable predictive of appointment-keeping is the client's prior appointment-keeping pattern. (b) Second in importance is age, baseline 50 years (clients under 50 kept 64.1% of their appointments, versus 80% by clients 50 or older). (c) Third in importance is appointment interval, with 81.5% of appointments kept for appointments less than 6 weeks apart and 72.6% appointments kept for appointments 6 weeks or more apart.

Limitations of Inference: The client sample used to generate the model is not described in detail, and the same site was used to test as well as develop the model. The model's generalizability to other sites needs to be tested.

6. DUPUIS, A. and others. Assessment of the psychological factors and responses in self-managed patients. _Diabetes Care_ 3(1):117-119, Jan-Feb 1980.

   Population Studied: 10 young adult and adolescent clients with insulin-dependent diabetes.

   Purpose: To determine whether a group program on blood glucose self-monitoring optimizes adherence, carbohydrate control, and emotional health.

   Design: 8 month study; random selection; no control or contrasting treatment group; pre- and post-test measures.

   Interventions: A peer instructor (a juvenile-onset diabetic in good control) led the group in weekly meetings. Initially, members received information about blood glucose self-monitoring, insulin injections, meal planning, etc. Members would share feelings about diabetes and its management. Over time, members relied less on instruction and more on each other for practical advice.

   Measures: (a) Depression; (b) Hba_1c "(blood glucose)" levels; (c) sense of mastery of disease.

   Results: (a) Initially, clients were quite depressed; after 8 months, they were significantly less depressed. (b) Clients' sense of mastery of their disease appeared to increase markedly by the end of 8 months. (the author attributes this to their frequent daily blood glucose tests: the more immediate feedback allowed clients to better calibrate diet, exericse, and insulin. The author also believes that self-monitoring reduced denial of the illness.) (c) Decreased HbA_1c "(blood glucose)" levels were noted.

   Limitations of Inference: Very small sample; no control group. Further research is needed to validate these case study findings.

7. EARP, J., and Ory, M. G. The effects of social support and health professional home visits on patient adherence to hypertension regimens. A paper presented at the 1979 National Conference on High Blood Pressure Control, Washington, D.C., April 6, 1979.

Population Studied: 218 clients with hypertension (50% had blood pressure less than 95mm Hg); 75% Black, middle-aged, poor, and poorly educated. The majority were from small towns or rural areas and were semi- or unskilled laborers; 35% of the males were unemployed. Clients faced financial and transportation barriers in keeping their clinic appointments.

Purpose: To test whether (a) active family participation in blood pressure monitoring and (b) home visits by health professionals are effective strategies for helping clients achieve greater adherence with their medical regimens.

Design: 18 month study; follow-up at 24 months; random assignment; 1 control group and 2 experimental groups.

Interventions: (a) Control group: routine medical care (not described). (b) Home visits: clients were visited an average of 3 times a year by either a pharmacist or visiting nurse; visits generally lasted 1 1/2 hours, with discussion of client and family concerns during first hour, hypertension specific discussion in last half hour. (c) Home visits and family support for self-monitoring: in addition to the home visits as in group b, clients and family were also instructed in blood pressure self-measurement.

Measures: Blood pressure.

Results: (a) Blood pressure declined for all 3 groups during the first 18 months of the study. The drop was greatest for the experimental groups and least for the control. The largest drop was seen among group c clients. (b) While home visits by health professionals seem to be effective, as seen by the significant drop between entry and 18 months blood pressure among group b clients, they seem to be more effective when clients' significant others are systematically included both in the home visits and between visits as blood pressure monitors. At 24 months, (6 months after visiting had ceased) only group c has sustained a statistically significant decline. Blood pressure for groups b and a rose to their highest point post-entry. It seems that once motivational reinforcement through periodic visits is no longer provided, earlier improvement in blood pressure control wavers or disappears altogether.

Limitations of Inference: (a) Authors note that staff visited the group b clients (with no family involvement in blood pressure monitoring) significantly more often than the group c clients; this may have elevated early findings of group b. (b) The population studied was unique in that many had to travel 60 or more miles to the clinic, which may have affected the response to home visits. (c) This, in addition to the demographic characteristics of the client population, suggests the importance of replication to test generalizability.

8. ETZWILER, D. D. Teaching allied health professionals about self-management. _Diabetes Care_, 3(1):121-123 Jan 1980.

> Population Studied: 75 clients with diabetes, outpatients treated at a medical center.
>
> Purpose: To examine the usefulness of telephone follow-up to increase client adherence with written contracts to do urine testing.
>
> Design: 2-week follow-up; random assignment; 1 control and 2 experimental groups (25 each).
>
> Interventions: (a) All clients contracted to do urine testing at home and send the results to the clinic 2 weeks later in exchange for a telephone conversation with a health professional to discuss the results; (b) half the experimental group received 1 reminder phone call; (c) the other half received 2 reminder phone calls.
>
> Measures: Adherence was measured by whether client mailed urine test results to the physician.
>
> Results: Contracts were adhered to by 52% of the clients receiving no phone calls, by 64% of those receiving 1 call, and by 80% of those receiving 2 phone calls.
>
> Limitations of Inference: The author does not discuss the form of the contract. No tests of significance were performed on the data. It would be useful to expand the follow-up beyond 2 weeks to evaluate the length of telephone contact impact.

9. FISHBACH, R., and others. The patient and practitioner as co-authors of the medical records. _Patient Counselling and Health Education_, 2 (1):1-5, First Quarter 1980.

> Population Studied: 20 clients with diabetes, hypertension, and/or congestive heart problems.
>
> Purpose: To determine if co-authoring the medical record can benefit both provider and client by improving communication and collaboration, with implications for adherence.
>
> Design: 1 year pilot project; convenience rather than random sample; no control group; single intervention; pre- and post-measures.
>
> Interventions: The Problem Oriented Medical Record (POMR) matrix was used for mutual teaching and negotiation during all client visits. Each client was asked to formulate a problem list from his or her own perspective. The provider suggested

modifications, if needed, before the list was placed in the medical record. At each visit, client and provider co-authored a continuation note including symptoms, clinical findings, and assessment. A mutually acceptable plan was tailored specifically to the needs and lifestyle of the client. The plan functioned as a contract, describing the obligations and responsibilities of each. Patients kept a copy of the co-authored report, which they brought to all visits. The record also contained flow sheets of physiological data, home monitoring records, and relevant educational materials.

Measures: (a) Appointment keeping; (b) client perceptions of the record-sharing experiment.

Results: (a) Appointment keeping improved markedly. (b) There seemed to be fewer client misconceptions, and reduced client diffidence and passivity. Radical changes in clients' perception of roles or modes of interaction with health professionals did not occur immediately. As clients became more familiar with terminology and format, they began to focus on more relevant symptoms and became more articulate and effective historians.

Limitations of Inference: Since this was a pilot study, a small nonrandom sample of 20 clients was used. There was no control group or contrasting intervention against which to compare the outcomes of joint medical record authoring. The measures used are not described in enough detail to evaluate their validity or reliability. No statistical analysis was done.

10. GLANZ, K., and others. Linking research and practice in patient education for hypertension--patient responses to four educational interventions. Medical Care 19(2):141-152, Feb 1981.

Population Studied: 432 clients with hypertension; majority white, blue collar, and over 50; 57% had been diagnosed more than 5 years ago.

Purpose: To examine (a) how clients react to different educational interventions; and (b) how their reactions are related to changes in adherence behaviors.

Design: 1-3 month follow-up; random assignment (fully crossed design); no control group; 4 experimental groups, with subdivisions--1) written message, 2) phone call, 3) self-monitoring through record keeping, 4) social support; pre- and post-test measures.

Interventions: (a) Written message: half of these clients received written materials containing high-threat information regarding hypertension and its control, and half received a positive message. (b) Phone call: clients received a letter notifying them that a nurse from the study would call; the nurse called clients to ask about their regimens and blood pressure levels, and provided verbal reinforcement for any regimens that clients were trying to follow. (c) Self-monitoring: half of these clients kept a 14-day record of daily medications, side effects, and other adherence behaviors; the other half recorded their blood pressure daily. (d) Social support: a nurse met individually with clients and a social support person of the client's choice to develop a plan for enlisting the support person's help with some aspect of the client's regimen.

Measures: (a) Knowledge; (b) medication adherence; (c) adherence to diet. (Adherence measured by client self-report and pharmacy and medical record reviews.)

Results: There were no clear long term effects from the 4 interventions. However, the cuff self-monitoring group showed the greatest increase in adherence.

Limitations of Inference: The authors report that clients were fairly adherent to begin with and for that reason it may have been difficult to show much impact on adherence. Unlike most hypertension adherence studies, no objective measure such as blood pressure was used. Self-report measures were primary source of information.

11. GO, H., and Becker, H. Reducing broken appointments in a primary care clinic. The Journal of Ambulatory Care Management :23-30, May 1979.

Population Studied: Clients who had missed appointments at an adult primary care clinic, University of Maryland at Baltimore; demographic information not provided. 400 clients in Phase I; 538 in Phase II.

Purpose: (a) To identify key factors in broken appointments; (b) to evaluate the effectiveness of various modes of intervention.

Design: Phase I: duration unclear; random assignment; 1 control, 3 experimental groups (100 each). Phase II: 69 day study; 1 intervention to all clients for 7 days; remaining 62 days without the intervention served as control.

Intervention: Phase I: After-the-fact interventions--(a) nothing (control group). (b) phone calls inquiry and invitation to make new appointment. (c) post card, same invitation. (d) phone call and postcard. Phase II: Anticipatory intervention: for 7 days postcards were sent to all clients a few days before the scheduled appointment, giving time, date, and a phone number to call in case of a problem.

Measures: Appointment keeping.

Results: Phase I: (a) contacting clients after a missed
appointment did not significantly reduce missing later
appointments. Phase II: contact before an appointment did
significantly reduce missed appointments. (b) A regression
analysis determined that the active intervention strategy (i.e.,
postcard reminders) was effective in reducing the number of
irretrievable appointments by 38.7%.

Limitations of Inference: Since demographic information is not
provided, generalizability of results cannot be certain.

12. HAYNES, R. B. and others. Improvement of medication compliance in
    uncontrolled hypertension. The Lancet (1):1265-1268, Jun 1976.

Population Studied: 38 male steelworkers who had uncontrolled
hypertension and were nonadherent to therapy.

Purpose: To examine whether a set of behaviorally-oriented
strategies could enhance adherence.

Design: 1 year study; stratified assignment; control group (18)
and 1 experimental group (20).

Interventions: Control group received no new interventions.
Experimental group: (a) Clients were taught self-measurement of
blood pressure and encouraged to monitor routinely at home. (b)
They recorded daily medication and blood pressure on charts
illustrating their blood pressure goals. (c) They met with the
experimenters to review their daily habits and establish a
complementary medication routine. (d) In addition, they
reported for blood pressure checks every 2 weeks; at these
visits they received positive reinforcement for decreased blood
pressure and monetary credit towards ownership of the home
sphygmomanometer and stethoscope.

Measures: (a) Adherence to medication as measured by pill
counts; (b) blood pressure.

Results: (a) After 6 months, adherence among the experimental
clients exceeded adherence in the control group and their own
pre-study adherence by more than 20%. These differences were
statistically significant. (b) Adherence improvements among
experimental clients were paralleled by decreases in diastolic
blood pressure. Blood pressures fell in 17 of 20 experimental
clients (to goal, in 6 clients) and in 10 of 18 control
clients. Among the experimental group, the total decrease of
11-6 mm Hg approached the 13-2 mm Hg average observed among
highly adherent clients at 6 months.

Limitations of Inference: According to the authors,
self-monitoring clients received more attention than did clients
in the control, and this extra attention may have caused the
differences, rather than the nature of the interventions. The
authors point out that more research is needed to clarify this.

13. HEFFERIN, E. A. Health goal setting: Patient-nurse collaboration at
    Veterans Administration facilities. Military Medicine
    144(12):814-822, Dec 1979.

      Population Studied: 572 clients with a range of educational
levels, drawn from inpatient, outpatient, surgery, psychiatric,
and clinic care units at 6 VA hospitals.

      Purpose: To explore the effects of contracts on health
progress, client responsibility for treatment, and satisfaction
of client and nurse.

      Design: Duration of study not given; random assignment; 1
control and 1 experimental group.

      Interventions: (a) Control group: routine care with health
goals identified by nurses; (b) experimental group: clients
worked with nurses to develop contracts with both short and long
term goals.

      Measures: (a) Increments of health progress were estimated by
nurses on a 5-point scale for each health goal identified in the
client's contract. These assessments were made at weekly
intervals (or, for clinic clients, at scheduled return visits).
(b) Client and nurse satisfaction with care were measured
through a 20-item questionnaire.

      Results: (a) Clients who developed contracts showed more and
faster health progress, according to nurse ratings, than did
clients who did not develop contracts. (b) They also showed
significantly more satisfaction with involvement in their care
than did the control clients. (c) Nurses' satisfaction with
specific aspects of the care progress was higher when working
with the contracting clients than with the clients receiving
routine care.

      Limitations of Inference: Progress toward health goals was
determined by nurse's subjective assessment. Since inter-rater
reliability of this assessment was not reported, it is unclear
how consistent these ratings were between nurses. It seems
likely that nurses knew which clients had developed contracts
and that this could have introduced unconscious bias into their
assessment of client's progress; this problem is not addressed.

14. HERJE, P. Behavioral contracting with persons with low back pain: An experimental study. Masters Thesis, University of Wisconsin-Madison, 1981.

   Population Studied: 60 clients with low back pain; outpatient setting, 29 males, 31 females; aged 16-78.

   Purpose: To examine the short term effectiveness of patient education plus behavioral contracting compared to patient education alone.

   Design: 2 week study; random assignment; 1 control group (30); 1 experimental group with nurse (30); pre- and post-treatment tests.

   Interventions: (a) Control groups received an interactive, programmed audiovisual instruction in one educational session with no contracting; (b) contract groups received the same educational session and afterwards negotiated a written behavioral contract on how he or she could implement the material just reviewed about back care.

   Measures: (a) Self-reported low back exercises and protective postures, (b) low back knowledge, (c) reported pain and medication usage.

   Results: (a) The contracting group reported doing more low back exercises and more protective postures than the control group, (b) there were no significant differencess between the groups in knowledge scores, (c) there were no significant differences in reported pain or medication usage.

   Limitations of Inference: A relatively short follow-up time was used to evaluate impact, suggesting the need for longer term follow-up in future studies. It would be useful to validate self-report with observable measures of health status or adherence.

15. IRSIGLER, K., and Bali-Taubald, C. Self-monitored blood glucose: the essential feedback signal in the diabetic patient's effort to achieve normoglycemia. Diabetes Care 3(1):163-170, Jan-Feb 1980.

   Population Studied: 17 pregnant women with diabetes.

   Purpose: To evaluate the effectiveness of a home blood glucose self-monitoring program in helping clients achieve normoglycemia.

   Design: Duration not indicated; comparison to past records of 4 similar clients is only control.

   Interventions: (a) Clients met in small groups for 1-1 1/2 hours weekly, led by a physician, a psychologist, and a dietician. At each session, one topic (e.g., diet, hypoglycemia) was presented, and individual problems of metabolic control were discussed in detail. (b) Clients also learned to self-monitor their blood glucose using Eyetone reflectance meters or Reflomats. They kept 24-hour profiles of insulin, food intake, and glucose levels. (d) Clients were closely supervised and seen weekly in the clinic throughout pregnancy.

Measures: (a) Blood glucose levels; (b) number of days of hospitalization. Records of 4 clients from an earlier intensive care group, for whom day-long profiles under outpatient conditions were available, were matched for White classification and week of pregnancy with profiles from the self-monitoring group.

Results: (a) Comparison of blood glucose profiles showed significantly better control (with near normal glycemia) in the self-monitoring group than in the earlier group of clients. (b) There were 45 fewer necessary days of hospitalization as compared to the earlier group of clients. (c) Clients were enthusiastic about the program.

Limitations of Inference: The authors point out that pregnant women, being highly motivated, represented an ideal group of clients, both for examining the suitability of the method and making the criteria of quality of control as strict as possible. Since there was no real control group and the sample studied was small, there is a need to replicate the study.

16. JOHNSON, A. and others. Self-recording of blood pressure in the management of hypertension. Canadian Medical Association Journal 119:1034-1039, Nov 4, 1978.

   Population Studied: 136 clients, men and women aged 35-65 with uncontrolled hypertension.

   Purpose: To test whether client self-monitoring of blood pressure augmented by home visits increases adherence and blood pressure control.

   Design: 6 month study; random assignment; 1 control group (34) and 3 experimental groups; pre- and post-measurement.

   Interventions: Control group received regular clinic blood pressure checks. 3 experimental groups: (a) Clients received monthly home visits by a staff person who measured and recorded blood pressure; (b) Clients received a blood pressure kit and instruction in self-recording; they kept charts of their daily readings, which they brought along to clinic visits; (c) Clients monitored their own blood pressures and received monthly home visits to measure blood pressure.

Measures: (a) Blood pressure; (b) adherence, as measured by client self-report and pill counts.

Results: After 6 months: (a) all groups showed similar reduction in diastolic blood pressure; (b) adherence appeared to improve more among subjects doing self-monitoring, but not significantly; (c) the interventions did not affect clients who said they had no trouble remembering to take their medication, but did prove beneficial for clients who said they had such a problem; (d) among the self-monitoring groups, those who received home visits recorded their blood pressure significantly more often.

Limitations of Inference: Only limited demographic information is provided.

17. LEVINE, D., and others. Health education for hypertensive patients. JAMA 241(16):1700-1703, Apr 1979.

Population Studied: 400 hypertensives; 91% Black, 76% female; urban; low income; mean age of 54 years.

Purpose: To compare the separate and combined effectiveness of 3 educational interventions on client adherence and blood pressure control.

Design: 18 month study; sequential, randomized, factorial design; 1 control group, 8 combinations of 3 interventions; pre- and post-measures.

Interventions: 3 interventions, singly and in combinations. (a) Exit interview: 20-minute interview with client at clinic after routine visit, answering client questions and tailoring the regimen. (b) Home visit: visited at home, the client identified a household member expected to provide the most adherence reinforcement; this person was given a separate interview and specific information on hypertension, what the client could do, how the person could help client adherence and the importance of medications even when the client felt fine. (c) Small group: a series of three 2-hour group sessions, led by a social worker, helped members to assess their personal needs, establish a contract of expectations with the leader, practice problem-solving as a group, develop skills through role playing, and monitor each other's blood pressure.

Measures: (a) Blood pressure; (b) adherence to medication; (c) weight change; (d) appointment keeping.

Results: (a) Except for the exit alone condition all interventions (singly or in combination) demonstrated some improvement in blood pressure over the control group. The percentage of clients who achieved blood pressure control increased 28% among clients assigned to all 3 interventions (38% of clients pre-intervention vs 66% of clients post-intervention had controlled blood pressure). Combinations of any 2 interventions had a modest but positive effect. Of single interventions, 18% more of the small-group clients and 11% more of the home visit/family support achieved control. The combined condition of exit interview + home visit showed greatest improvement in medication adherence (53% reporting high adherence, 13% reporting low, vs. 40% and 20% in the control group). (c) Clients with the exit interview as a single intervention did best at weight reduction, with 56% losing at least 2 kg (vs. 35% in the control group). (d) Increased appointment keeping was seen with home visit/family support clients (to 76%), with home visit and exit interview combined (to 75%), and with exit interview and small groups combined (to 73%); control group appointment keeping was at 63%.

Limitations of Inference: Demographic characteristics may limit generalizability. Almost half of the clients assigned to the small-group intervention did not participate; this self-selection process may bias the small-group findings. The random assignment of clients to interventions resulted in an unequal percentage of clients with controlled blood pressure assigned to the various intervention conditions. Only 34% of the clients started out with controlled blood pressure who received the small group and no other intervention. In contrast, 45% of the clients started out with controlled blood pressure who received the exit interview and family support home visit. The authors do try to standardize this through an "effectiveness index" they developed.

18. LORIG, K., and others. A randomized, prospective, controlled study of the effects of health education for people with arthritis. American Rheumatism Association Meetings, June 1981.

Population Studied: 309 individuals with arthritis; mean age of 67; drawn from the community.

Purpose: To examine how a group educational intervention affects behaviors and health outcomes.

Design: 18 month follow-up; random assignment of volunteers; 1 experimental group; 1 control; pre- and post-measure.

Interventions: (a) Individuals participated in 6 weekly 2 hour educational group sessions led by 2 trained lay leaders. After presenting didactic material in the first quarter of the class, participants broke into dyads or small groups to apply the principles to their own situation, e.g. to develop their own exercise plan given their personal strength, flexibility, and time constraints. At the end of the class, participants returned to the large group to summarize their own plans. (b) Individuals on a waiting list for the educational group sessions acted as a control group.

Measures: 1) Reported pain; 2) amount of walking; 3) number of physician visits; 4) amount spent on medications.

Results: 1) Preliminary analysis of 8 month follow-up data indicated the educational group (EG) participants reported a 20% decrease in pain, with no change in the control group. 2) EG participants increased the frequency of walking 4 blocks or more by 3-5 times a month while controls decreased by 2.3 times per month. 3) the EG participants decreased their annual visits to physicians an average of 1.5 visits, twice the amount for the control group. 4) There were no detected changes in the amount spent on medications.

Preliminary analysis of 20 month follow-up data for the 200 individuals who remained in the study indicates that pain, disability and physician visit rates declined even further from 8 month levels.

Limitations of Inference: Little demographic data is presented.

19. MORISKY, D., and others. The relative impact of health education for low- and high-risk patients with hypertension. Preventive Medicine 9:550-558, 1980. (See Levine, D., Green, L., et. al. for a description of the same study.)

Population Studied: 400 hypertensives, 91% Black, 76% female with a median age of 54 years.

Purpose: To analyze the effects of an educational program on a group of hypertensive patients comparing those with known higher risk of stroke and heart attack with a group whose risks were believed to be lower.

Design: 18 months; a randomized (2X2X2) factorial design with assignment to 3 interventions--1) exit interview, 2) home visit, and 3) small groups; pre- and post-tests.

Results: (a) Educational interventions were equally effective for promoting adherence among high risk and low risk clients. (b) Both lower- and higher-risk clients had similar appointment keeping ratios of about 66%. (c) Clients at lower risk increased in blood pressure control from any single or combination of interventions. The high risk clients only benefited from certain interventions and the benefits were usually less than for the lower-risk group. For high risk

clients the greatest increase in percentage of clients with
controlled blood pressure occurred for two groups--First, the
clients who received a home visit for family support from 26%
clients pre-visit to 48% clients post-visit achieved control
representing a 22% percentage point increase; and second, the
high risk clients who received all three interventions--exit
interview, family home visit, and small group resulting in a 27%
percentage point increase in clients with controlled blood
pressure. The authors recommend that for high-risk clients, the
stronger and more complex interventions be used (family home
visit and small group) whereas the exit interview can be used
with low risk clients.

Limitations of Inference: (See Levine and others, 1979.)

20. NESSMAN, D., and others. Increasing compliance in patient-operated
    hypertension groups. Archives of Internal Medicine 140:1427-1430,
    Nov 1980.

    Population Studied: 51 men and 1 woman with inadequately
    controlled hypertension; mean age 55 years; 5 Black, 8
    Mexican-American, and 39 White.

    Purpose: To evaluate a self-management training program for
    hypertensive clients.

    Design: 8 month study; random assignment; 1 control and 1
    experimental group (26 each); pre- and post-test measures.

    Interventions: All clients were seen weekly for 8 weeks. (a)
    Clients assigned to the control group received regular medical
    treatment at a nurse-operated hypertension clinic, and listened
    to audiotaped hypertension information. (b) Clients in the
    experimental group met in a group; clinicians sought to create
    an atmosphere of client responsibility and informed
    decision-making through an individually tailored education
    program, discussion, and self-help approach. Information on
    hypertension and medications (including side effects) was given
    at the level desired by group participants. Participants
    discussed perception of disease as serious, personal
    susceptibility, belief in and satisfaction with the treatment.
    Clients learned to take their own blood pressure and formulated
    their own regimen within the framework of standard diet and drug
    protocols.

    Measures: (a) Blood pressure; (b) pill counts, and (c)
    attendance.

    Results: (a) At the end of 6 months the mean systolic and
    diastolic blood pressure of both experimental and control groups
    decreased significantly. The decrease in blood pressure was

significantly greater for the experimental than for the control group. (b) Attendance and pill counts were significantly better for the experimental than for the control group.

Limitations of Inference: Only 10.4% of the noncompliant, hypertensives contacted for the study agreed to participate, so it is likely that a self-selection process occurred. Since control clients were seen weekly, it is likely that this additional attention resulted in blood pressure decreases for the control group.

21. OGBUOKIRI, J. E. Self-monitoring of blood pressure in hypertensive subjects and its effects on patients compliance. Drug Intelligence and Clinical Pharmacy 14:424-427, Jun 1980.

Population Studied: 24 clients with hypertension; low-income aged 27-58; 95% Black, 85% women.

Purpose: To test the hypothesis that clients who monitor their own blood pressure are more adherent than those who do not.

Design: 5 month study; random assignment; 1 control group (12), 1 experimental group (12); pre- and post-measurement of blood pressure, post-measurement of adherence.

Interventions: (a) Both groups received routine care: they were presented with information by a pharmacist, and a tape-recorded program and pamphlets concerning hypertension, its management, and the importance of adherence to the therapeutic regimen. (b) Experimental group: clients were also instructed about taking and recording their own blood pressures at home.

Measures: (a) Blood pressure; (b) weight; (c) medication-taking, as measured by pill counts, prescription refills, and self-report.

Results: (a) There was no difference in blood pressure between the 2 groups: blood pressure increased slightly for both. (b) There was no difference in weight loss: both groups lost weight slightly. (c) The percentage of adherent clients rose from 38% to 73% in the self-monitoring group and from 32% to 59% in the control group.

Limitations of Inference: (a) Small sample. (b) The baseline systolic blood pressure of the control group was 126 mm Hg; for the self-monitoring group it was 129 mm Hg. Given these values, it would be difficult for any intervention to result in a dramatic reduction of blood pressure.

22. PETERSON, C. M., and others. Feasibility of improved blood glucose control in patients with insulin-dependent diabetes mellitus. Diabetes Care 2:329-335, Jul-Aug 1979.

Population Studied: 10 clients with severe insulin-dependent diabetes of approximately 10 years duration; average age 25.

Purpose: To evaluate a self-management program for diabetics designed to optimize adherence and carbohydrate control.

Design: 8 month study; no control group; during- and post-intervention measures.

Interventions: Clients met weekly in group meetings with a diabetic group leader and were seen monthly in the clinic by physicians who were available on a 24-hour basis by means of a beeper call system. Clients learned to measure their own blood glucose using a blood glucose meter. They kept diaries of urinary and blood sugar testing and insulin dosage. Their insulin regimens were adjusted to a spilt-dose schedule. In addition, clients were taught to exercise at a sports training institute, following a general 35-minute routine that included warm-ups, pedaling on an ergometer bicycle, and weight training. Each exercise was performed individually with a trainer. No attempt was made to adjust exercise time to meals, but clients tested their blood sugars before and after the workouts.

Another aspect of the program involved clients' learning to calibrate food and insulin, and to experiment with different types of food. They were made aware of the necessity of meal planning and encouraged to keep food intake records.

Measures: 1) Blood glucose levels; 2) blood pressure; 3) resting pulse rates; 4) body fat; 5) body weight; 6) hospitalization; 7) drop-out rates; 8) adherence to exercise; 9) alkaline phosphatase levels; 10) nerve condition values. These measures were evaluated after 3 and 8 months.

Results: After three months, 1) there was a significant decrease in blood glucose levels. 2) The mean systolic blood pressure decreased by over 10 mm Hg and remained at the low value. 3) The mean resting pulse rate dropped from 82 to 70 per minute. 4) Mean body fat dropped from 19% to 14%. 5) Weight did not change significantly. 6) There were 7 hospitalizations related to diabetes in the group during the year prior to the study; during the 3-month study period there were none. 7) None of the clients dropped out of treatment. 8) Clients kept to the regular exercise program 82% of the time. 9) Alkaline phosphatase levels decreased in each client as blood glucose control improved. 10) 3 of the 7 clients with nerve conduction abnormalities at the beginning of the study showed a return to normal values; 1 of these 3 clients improved dramatically.

> Limitations of Inference: In this study, clients were not randomly selected but, rather, they were referred by their physicians. No control group of clients was followed for comparative purposes. The sample size was quite small. There is a strong need for study replication.

23. SACCONE, A. The effects of experimenter versus significant other-controlled reinforcement and choice of target behavior on weight loss. Behavior Therapy 9:271-278, 1978.

> Population Studied: 48 women and 1 man, mean age of 37, ranging from 16-100% overweight (mean=45.8%).

> Purpose: To assess the degree to which targeting eating behaviors rather than weight loss goals and involving a significant other as a reinforcing agent would enhance the effectiveness of a stimulus-control weight loss program.

> Design: Duration of study unstated; random assignment to 1 of 6 interventions based on percentage of overweight--(1) program only monitoring weight and behavior; (2) program with reinforcement by therapist for weight loss; (3) program with reinforcement by therapist for eating behavior change; (4) program with reinforcement by significant other for weight loss; or (5) program with reinforcement by significant other for eating behavior change. No treatment control group.

> Interventions: All treatment groups met for eight 1-hour group sessions for 9 weeks. (1) Program only group constitutes the basic stimulus-control package given to all active treatment conditions. Clients were taught how to monitor food intake, to control individual and environmental cues to eating, to establish nutritionally sound diets, and to increase exercise above baseline levels. (2) In addition the reinforcement group received monetary reinforcement for weight loss from the therapist during the last 6 weeks of the program. (3) This group was reinforced by the therapist for eating behavior change (clients monitored their eating habits at the dinner meal on a 9-point checklist and received monetary reinforcement for appropriate eating behavior). (4) This group was reinforced by a significant other for weight loss, usually by a spouse who attended the third group session to learn to monitor and record the client's weight every day and pay the client once a week according to reinforcement. (5) This group was reinforced by a significant other for good eating habits by monitoring the client's eating behavior on the same checklist used by the Therapist-Behavior Group. (6) No-treatment contol group.

Measures: Weight change.

Results: Rewards by a significant other had a stronger positive
impact than did rewards by a therapist. Reinforcement of eating
habits resulted in significantly more weight loss than did
reinforcement of weight lost. Each of the 5 active treatment
groups demonstrated significant weight losses, while the
No-Treatment Group displayed a nonsignificant weight gain.
Participation in active treatment produced significantly greater
weight loss than no treatment supporting the hypothesis that the
basic stimulus-control package is superior to no treatment.

Limitations of Inference: A relatively small number of clients
participated in each of the interventions although a total of 49
persons were in the study. The study included only 1 male, so
it would be important to replicate the study with males. Since
the time of the post-test weight measurement is unclear it would
be important to clarify how long the positive effects of the
interventions last.

24. SCHULMAN, B. A. Active patient orientation and outcomes in
    hypertension treatment. Medical Care 17(3):267-279, Mar 1979.

Population Studied: 99 hypertensive clients being served in 2
hypertension clinics, one in a VA hospital and the other in a
university hospital. (The same population used by Steckel,
1977).

Purpose: To investigate the relationship between clients'
perceptions that they have been actively involved in their care
and the desired outcomes of treatment.

Design: 18 month study; random assignment; 1 control group and
2 experimental groups; pre- and post-measures.

Interventions: (a) All received routine care; (b) both
experimental groups received counseling and 5 educational
booklets on hypertension; (3) one experimental group also
negotiated contracts with the clinic nurse.

Measures: (a) Client perceptions of involvement in their own
care, as measured by an Active Patient Orientation (APO)
questionnaire. (b) Reported adherence. (c) Client faith in the
treatment and belief that the visit had responded to their
needs. (d) Blood pressure.

Results: After 18 months: (a) Clients with contracts reported
more involvement as active participants in their treatment than
did non-contracting clients. (b) Clients who reported most
strongly that they had been involved in their care (whether they
had contracted or not) were more likely to report adherence,
believe in the treatment, feel that the visit had met their
needs, and have controlled blood pressure.

Limitations of Inference: The validity and reliability of the APO instrument used to measure clients' perceptions is not discussed in detail and therefore it is difficult to evaluate.

SCHULMAN, B.A. and M.A. SWAIN. "Active patient orientation." Patient Counseling and Health Education, First Quarter:32-37 (1980).

See SCHULMAN, 1979. This article is based on the same research.

25. STECKEL, S. B., and Swain, M. A. Contracting with patients to improve compliance. Hospitals 51:81-84, Dec 1977.

Population Studied: 115 hypertensive clients being served on an outpatient basis.

Purpose: To explore 2 means of improving client adherence--patient education and contingency contracting.

Design: 18 month study; random assignment; 1 control group and 2 experimental groups; pre- and post-measures.

Interventions: (a) All clients received routine care; (b) both experimental groups also received counseling, and educational booklets on hypertension; (c) one experimental group also negotiated contracts with the clinic nurse.

Measures: (a) Knowledge (written test); (b) drop-out rate; (c) appointment keeping; (d) blood pressure.

Results: (a) Post-test knowledge scores of the contracting counseling and education group were significantly higher than those of the noncontracting counseling and education group. (b) 7.9% of the routine care group was lost from treatment, 35.9% of the noncontracting counseling and education (control) group was lost from treatment, and none of the contracting counseling and education group was lost from treatment. (c) There were 5 missed appointments in the control group, 11 for the noncontracting group, and no missed appointments in the contracting group. (d) Diastolic blood pressures for the contracting group were under clinical control by the second visit and remained so; no consistent picture of blood pressure control was presented by the other groups.

Limitations of Inference: Although the clients were randomly assigned to treatment groups, no data is provided on their baseline blood pressures. Owing to loss of clients, the control and noncontracting counseling and education groups, no statistical analysis could be done beyond the fourth clinic appointment.

SWAIN, M.A. and S.B. STECKEL. "Influencing adherence among hypertensives," Research in Nursing and Health, 4:213-222 (1981).

See STECKEL and SWAIN, 1977. This article is based on the same research.

26. STECKEL, S. B., and Swain, M. A. Increasing adherence of outpatients to therapeutic regimens. Project Final Report, 1981.

Population Studied: 379 outpatient clients with hypertension, diabetes mellitus, or rheumatoid arthritis; average age 53, clients had condition for an average of 10.5 years.

Purpose: To determine the effectiveness of written behavioral contracts to increase client participation in health-related behaviors and to increase adherence to therapeutic regimens.

Design: 3-year follow-up; random assignment; 1 control group, 1 experimental; pre- and post-measures.

Interventions: (a) All clients received routine care with the same number of visits and type of staff emotional support; (b) clients in the experimental group negotiated contracts with a nurse.

Measures: (a) Missed appointments; (b) weight; (c) for diabetes, fasting blood glucose; (d) blood pressure.

Results: (a) The contracting group had significantly fewer missed appointments and significantly more weight loss; (b) for diabetics, there was no difference between the contracting and noncontracting groups in their fasting blood levels; (c) blood pressure was significantly lower for the contracting group. The data for clients with arthritis was not yet analyzed thoroughly.

Limitations of Inference: According to the authors, fasting blood sugar is an inaccurate measure of adherence. Some non-adherent clients fast prior to the measurement enough that their readings are comparable to those of adherent clients.

27. SYME, S. Drug treatment of mild hypertension: social and psychological considerations. Annals New York Academy of Sciences, 1978.

Population Studied: 244 clients with hypertension; 85% black, 90% medically indigent.

Purpose: To see if clients receiving outreach home visits would be more successful in hypertension control after 7 months than clients not receiving outreach.

Design: 7 month study; random assignment to 2 experimental groups and 1 control (group size not stated); pre- and post-measures.

Interventions: (a) All clients received routine medical care from the clinic staff at regular intervals. One group received routine care alone. (b) One group of clients also attended weekly meetings led by a health educator and nurse at the clinic for 12 weeks, participants were taught the seriousness of hypertension, personal susceptibility to organ damage, possibility of side effects, the physician's approach to treatment and efficacy of treatment. (c) In addition to routine care 1 set of clients received home visits by a community health worker recruited from the target community and given intensive 1 month training.

Measures: 1) Blood pressure; 2) adherence (measure not described).

Results: 1) More clients receiving home visits had controlled diastolic blood pressure than either the clients in routine care or weekly meetings did. The difference in proportion under control was 23% between home visits and clients in routine care; and 7% between home visits and weekly meetings. 2) Good compliers in the outreach group were twice as successful in controlling diastolic blood pressure as good compliers attending weekly small group meetings. 55% of the home visit group were judged compliant with medications whereas only 41% of the clients in the group approach were so judged. The authors hypothesize home visits helps to reduce client stress thereby contributing to blood pressure control.

Limitations of Inference: Only preliminary data analysis is reported. No information is given about pre-intervention blood pressure and aside from percentage changed, no data on blood pressure values post-intervention are given. The author does not indicate how they judged whether clients were "compliant."

28. TAKALA, J., and others. Improving compliance with therapeutic regimens in hypertensive patients in a community health center. Circulation 59(3):540-543, Mar 1979.

Population Studied: 202 rural hypertensives in Finland, median age 51.5, not under treatment at start of study.

Purpose: To examine whether simple rearrangements of health education and organization can improve adherence with therapeutic regimen.

Design: 1 year study; random assignment; 1 control and 1 experimental group.

Interventions: (a) All clients received routine care; (b) experimental group also received a follow-up card with recorded blood pressure readings taken during the visit to the health center, medication prescribed, and the exact time of the next visit.

Measures: Blood pressure.

Results: (a) 3 persons out of 78 (4%) dropped out of experimental group, 16 of 86 (19%) dropped out of control group. The difference was statistically significant (p 0.01). (b) Desired blood pressure level was achieved by 63 (81%) of the experimental group and 55 (64%) of the control group.

Limitations of Inference: Cultural differences may reduce generalizability of results to U.S. populations.

29. UREDA, J. R. The effect of contract witnessing on motivation and weight loss in a weight control program. Health Education Quarterly 7(3):163-185, Fall 1980.

Population Studied: 106 overweight volunteers (98 women and 8 men).

Purpose: To investigate the influence of commitment as an important factor in a behavioral contract for a weight control program.

Design: 4 week intervention with follow-up at 4 months; 1 control and 1 experimental group (53 each).

Interventions: (a) All clients took part in a 4 week, 8 hour behavioral self-management and educational program. Each client received, read, signed, and returned 3 behavioral-intention contracts to the instructor. The contracts involved program participation, completion of a nutrition education notebook, and establishment of a weight-controlling routine. These contracts addressed 4 different dimensions: 1) a goal statement; 2) a statement of volition and self-responsibility; 3) a statement on belief in the consistency of the contract objectives with the achievement and maintenance of the desired weight loss goal; and 4) a commitment statement signed by the client. (b) The experimental (enhanced commitment) group also had a relative or friend witness and sign the contract.

Measures: (a) Weight loss; (b) behavioral intentions, as measured on a post-test questionnaire for which clients specified (on a 1-7 scale) the probability that they would perform 16 behaviors to influence weight loss (e.g., exercising regularly, controlling portions).

Results: (a) The enhanced commitment group showed significantly stronger intentions 10 to 15 weeks after contracting to perform behaviors conductive to weight loss; (b) the enhanced commitment group of clients lost weight at a significantly faster rate than the control group of clients.

Limitations of Inference: The study does not follow the clients long enough to determine if their target weight loss goals were actually achieved, or if the clients were able to maintain their weight loss.

30. WEBB, P. Effectiveness of patient education and psychosocial counseling in promoting compliance and control among hypertensive patients. Journal of Family Practice 10(6):1047-1055, 1980.

Population Studied: 123 hypertensive clients; low income, rural, Black.

Purpose: To examine whether additional patient education or additional psychosocial counseling would improve compliance or blood pressure control significantly better than regular family physician visits alone.

Design: 3 month study with follow-up at 18 months; random assignment; 1 control, 2 experimental groups; pre- and post-test measures.

Interventions: (a) All clients had regular physician visits. (b) The education group also had 3 group sessions by a trained nurse health educator, spaced 1 month apart and each lasting 1 hour; each session included the patient learner in group discussion in which the group openly voted on what new behaviors they would endorse and adopt. (c) The psychosocial counseling group had 3 individual counseling sessions with a trained social worker; each session lasted 1 hour, with 3 weeks between sessions. Counseling sessions focused on the problems of individual clients as identified by the client. 10 minutes of every session were devoted to muscle relaxation training.

Measures: (a) Blood pressure, (b) appointment keeping, (c) medication adherence.

Results: Follow-up appointment keeping rates did not differ significantly between the groups. Blood pressure improved in all 3 groups, with the rate of improvement greatest in the educational group. Neither education nor psychosocial counseling groups showed a significantly greater increase in medication adherence or diastolic blood pressure control than did the control group.

Limitations of Inference: It seems possible that the monthly contact with the physician for 3 months may have been in itself a significant treatment.

31. WYKA, C. A., and others. Group education for the hypertensive. Cardiovascular Nursing 16(1):1-5, Jan-Feb 1980.

Population Studied: 33 ambulatory male hypertensives who were being treated with no more than 3 drugs; who expressed an interest in the group educational program; and were without documented complications of hypertension.

Purpose: To measure the effectiveness of hypertensive group education on knowledge gained and change in health behavior.

Design: 3 month study; no control group; pre- and post-test.

Interventions: 3 groups met 1 1/2 hours weekly for 5 weeks. Clients were encouraged to bring a significant other to each session. Group leaders attempted to cultivate 1) a feeling of acceptance and security as part of a group sharing a common concern; 2) active involvement in the process of sharing common fears, perceptions and attitudes with a homogeneous group; 3) a great commitment to integrate knowledge into behavior. Multidisciplinary education included complications, medications, special diets, exercise, and clinical follow-up.

Measures: (a) Self-reported change in exercise, stress reduction, smoking behavior; (b) blood pressure.

Results: Those patients with poor to low pre-outcome behavior scores before the course tended to score better and have the largest change in the post-test than those with higher pre-outcome behavior scores prior to classes. Patients with greater number of risk factors demonstrated more improvement in their behavioral outcome than those with fewer risk factors. The most affected area in post-outcome behavior was the lowering of blood pressure to normal range. Another behavioral outcome which was strikingly altered was exercise.

Limitations of Inference: No control group, males only, small sample size, all suggest the need to replicate the findings.

32. ZIESAT, H. A. Behavior modification in the treatment of hypertension. International Journal of Psychiatry in Medicine 8(3):257-265, 1977-78.

Population Studied: 10 male clients with hypertension; average age 52, taking medication 4 times daily.

Purpose: To evaluate effectiveness of a behavior modification program as an addition to medical treatment for blood pressure control.

Design: 3-week measurement; random assignment; 1 control group (5) and 1 experimental group (5); pre- and post-measure.

Interventions: (a) Control group received only weekly blood pressure checks. (b) Experimental group attended 4 weekly group meetings where they received information on hypertension, chose an object or daily event to be used as a cue to take medication, learned to measure their own and each other's blood pressure, and chose a social ally (such as a close friend or spouse) to provide reinforcement for their regimens.

Measures: Blood pressure.

Results: Clients in the intervention group showed a significant decrease in blood pressure levels; no change was noted in the control group.

Limitations of Inference: The small all male sample with only short-term follow-up suggests the need for study replication with longer-term follow-up and a sample of both males and females.

AHA No. 070150

ISBN 0-87258-380